ENDORSI

In *Miraculous Identity*, Linda Breitman demystifies what it means to connect with God, to have a relationship with our Creator. Christians are often confounded by these concepts but are embarrassed to ask, "What does it really mean and how do I get there?" I am grateful that Linda has shown us how to cross the threshold of our human existence and enter the heavenly realms. Once you've experienced this kind of intimacy with God, you will want to keep coming back. Those moments with God have been life-changers for me.

Michele Rigby Assad, Former CIA Intelligence Officer and author of *Breaking Cover: My Secret Life in the CIA and What it Taught Me About What's Worth Fighting For*

This refreshing, timely book by Linda Breitman covers the full spectrum of our Christian life. It's not an ordinary book. It contains the matchless keys to become all God created you to be – to fulfill your destiny. As you integrate the principles taught into your daily life, you will walk in a new dimension of the Holy Spirit. I highly recommend *Miraculous Identity* as an invaluable source of encouragement to you.

Gary Oates, Author of *Open My Eyes, Lord*

Our salvation is miraculous! Kingdom is living beyond salvation and into the supernatural life of our new man and true Identity. Linda Breitman's book, *Miraculous Identity*, is an invitation to come into a deeper revelation of intimacy with the God. Linda mentors the reader as she cleverly presents principals and insights, with prayers and activations, any believer can grasp and appropriate into their lives. This is a must read for those hungering to live in His presence!

Maria Sainz, Red Seal Ministries, San Diego, CA

The framework used by Linda for this identity study series is simplicity at its best. No matter where you are in your Christian walk *Miraculous Identity* is for you. From personal study, small group study, all the way to a conference style with interactive events, this book will bring freedom. The still small voice of Holy Spirit will touch you through Linda's words and engaging the proclamations found within its pages will shatter unseen strongholds in your life.

Pastor Mike Ferry, Cornerstone Christian Fellowship, Redmond, OR, author of "*Making Disciples, Releasing into Ministry*"

I love Linda's approach in *Miraculous Identity*. We have been friends for years, and I have seen her walk out the very things she is teaching here. She meets things head on, lays it out in a direct, clear, and concise manner, and then positions you into activations that are so direct and compelling! There is no intimidation—anyone can go where she's gone. She helps you remove every barrier, every hindrance and all excuses. There is no reason not to progress in more of God. We have used Linda's first book *The Real You - Believing Your True Identity* in a study group at our church –and literally, lives were changed. Thank you, Linda, for your hard work and yielding to God's adventure in your life. It was for us.

Pastor Judy Ross, Cloud 9 Worship Center, San Diego, CA

Miraculous Identity takes the reader on a beautiful "river cruise" right into a 3D surround sound experience with the Trinity. Scripture commands us to "Come boldly to the throne of grace that we may find grace to help in time of need;" the exhortations and rich scriptural meditations provided in this book escorts one to the throne and increases understanding that we are destined to LIVE there! This heaven-bound journey delights the soul and will accelerate miraculous transformation in every passenger.

Pastor Claudia Porter, Torch Life Church, Denver, CO

Not only does this book encourage and teach us all to go deeper with God, Linda Breitman understands that words are creative. Her scripture declarations are prophetic "smart bombs" that renew our minds, strengthen our faith, and heal our damaged emotions. Great job!

Pastor Juanita Childress, Jubilee Legacy International,
Jubilee Christian Center, San Jose, California

Perfect for prison ministries, Bible studies and ministry schools! I have used Linda's identity teachings in my jail and prison ministry and the results are phenomenal! *Miraculous Identity* takes us even deeper in experiencing God more intimately!

Pastor Pat Winn,
Redeemed Ones Jail and Prison Ministry, Inc. Aurora, CO

Linda is one of those wonderful gifts that God has given to the body of Christ that not only teaches believers who they are in Christ, she is also a personal revelation herself of this truth. As you read this book, you will feel the freedom pouring over you, releasing the chains of condemnation from over your life.

Dr. Robert Cathers, Jr, Pastor, The Gathering Place, Simi, CA

Miraculous Identity causes vision, hope and intention to rise up within the reader, including me! Even though I know I have been transformed by these beautiful words of life over the forty-two years of extravagant pursuit of my Bridegroom King, I found myself strengthened and encouraged again as I read. The scripture says, "A well-spoken word at just the right time is like golden apples in settings of silver". This is one of those books written in the right season when God 's people must know who they are in HIM and who He is in them.

Linda does a superb job in imparting His identity very simply but powerfully that will miraculously change anyone who will believe and take the time to be diligent in establishing these revelatory truths into their foundation.

Be blessed abundantly as you are renewed, reformed and reidentified as 'one who belongs to the King'.

Billie Alexander, Limitless Realms Int'l Ministries,
San Diego, CA

Miraculous Identity is inspirational! Have you experienced a "watershed moment" in your life—that moment in time when your life changed and you knew that it would not ever be the same again? Linda Breitman will open your heart, soul and mind to a greater intimacy with God. This book can literally change your life. For people of faith or who are lost—it is a "must read". It is poignant, compelling and teaches you how to make that spiritual connection with God. I loved it and so will you.

Blanquita Cullum,
Veteran Broadcast Journalist and Former Governor,
United States Broadcasting Board of Governor

Miraculous Identity will radically shift your life! All who read this book will know who they are, whose they are, and the miracle of their spiritual DNA--all that is at their disposal as a chosen, cherished child of God! Full of Scripture and creatively interactive, you will experience security and joy even in life's hardest circumstances as you determine to live in the love and power of the Holy Spirit flowing naturally though you every day. Miraculous!

Nancy Stafford
Actress, Speaker, and Author of *The Wonder of His Love: A Journey into the Heart of God*

Published by Linda Breitman Ministries.
© 2018 by Linda Breitman

ISBN-13: 978-0-9894113-8-7

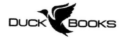

For information contact:
Linda Breitman Ministries
LindaBreitman.com

Miraculous
Identity

Unveiling Your Hidden Journey

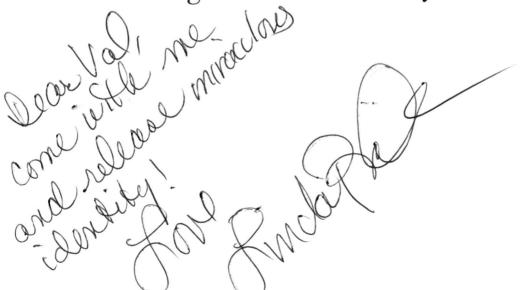

Dear Val,
come with me
and release miraculous
identity!
Love Linda R

Linda Breitman

I dedicate this book to my beloved husband, King Turkey! My grammar expert, wonderful advisor, and singer of my favorite song, "I love a duckie, quackie, quack, quack!"

He started living in heaven right after I started this book, yet his memory lives on in these pages.

Quack!

TO YOU ...
I AM GRATEFUL

To my book team: God brought me the best when He brought me YOU! Eden Gordon, Franciska Sore, and Suzy Lampe. I love you!

To my intercessors: You continually had my back! Pastor Mike Ferry, you were always available to me. John and Judy Ross and all of Cloud Nine Worship Center, your love is tangible. There are more people who prayed for me—too numerous to list. You know who you are—thank you for upholding me!

Eden Gordon of Eden Gordon Media has encouraged me, guided me, and laughed with me throughout the final stages of this book. I adore her. She is a gift from God. She is positive, uplifting, and is a woman of many talents. Now, she is going to have to put up with my humor for the rest of her life!

Franciska Sore, who resides in Croatia, is an amazing virtual assistant. You are extremely gifted and full of exotic, innovative ideas. I love that you are an out-of-the-box thinker.

Suzy has been at my right hand throughout this process. What a blessing. She even facetimes me to make sure I'm on track. You are a dear friend.

I am grateful to everyone who took the time to read the manuscript and write an endorsement for this book. Particularly, Gary Oates, who provided content feedback and editing. We had great discussions throughout! I highly value our friendship.

A special thanks to Alex Mooney, who was my excellent videographer. Our video shoots took longer than they should because we laughed so much all the way through. You are a blast!

I know there are many more who have stood with me and greatly impacted my life. I love you all and deeply appreciate you.

CONTENTS

FOREWORD

In *Miraculous Identity*, Linda Breitman demystifies what it means to connect with God, to have a relationship with our Creator. Christians are often confounded by these concepts but are embarrassed to ask, "What does it really mean and how do I get there?"

I am grateful that Linda has shown us how to cross the threshold of our human existence and enter the heavenly realms. She has provided a methodology for forging a powerful relationship with God. Instead of just alluding to the fact that we need to be more plugged-in with our Creator, she provides wonderfully creative ideas on how to make that happen. I pray that this book touches you as much as it has me, as you move closer to the most powerful force in the universe, the Spirit of our living God.

Once you've experienced this kind of intimacy with God, you will want to keep coming back. Those moments with God have been life-changers for me.

MICHELE RIGBY ASSAD
Former CIA Intelligence Officer and author of
Breaking Cover: My Secret Life in the CIA and
What it Taught Me About What's Worth Fighting For

M any of us desire to have a closer, more intimate relationship with God, whether we have professed Christ for five minutes or five decades. Why? Because we love God for all He has done for us, and we recognize our lives is a marathon not a sprint fraught with challenges from the devil.

That's why seizing the opportunities to recognize God's activity in our lives every day is so important. And this is why I was thrilled to read *Miraculous Identity* by Linda Breitman.

Miraculous Identity acts as a scriptural tour guide from the natural fallen world to the spiritual world of God. Chapters in the book address how we can deepen our faithfulness, our humility, and our trust in God.

Features that make *Miraculous Identity* extraordinary are its use of declarations, activations, prayer, and scripture. Linda stresses the significance of each chapter topic with an extensive list of relevant verses.

I especially appreciate the activations, which address common questions or doubts readers may have about the material. These activations will answer questions and overcome your doubts.

Many Christians struggle with converting new spiritual information into prayer and *Miraculous Identity* addresses this challenge with the "prayer" and "heavenly word" sections in each chapter. The prayer section is a sample prayer for the reader, and the heavenly word prayer is a corresponding prayer in the "voice" of our Father.

Miraculous Identity is a handbook for transforming our attitude toward God's place in our lives to overcome the challenges women face such as the death of a spouse or surviving a life-threatening illness. A widow and breast cancer survivor, Linda walks readers through her journey to a profound understanding of God's place in our lives.

The workbook provides an opportunity for personal reflection on our identity as men and women, so we can see ourselves as God sees us, rather than how the world sees us. The teachings and applications address everyday problems in an easy to understand yet miraculous way! This book is a winner!

MELANIE COLLETTE,
Radio Host, Washington, D.C.

*Eternal life means to know and experience you
as the only true God, and to know and experience
Jesus Christ, as the Son whom you have sent.*

JOHN 17:3 PASSION TRANSLATION.

INTRODUCTION

You can know God personally and intimately—and you can *experience* Him. He designed you to enjoy a deep, engaging relationship with Him. The problem is most of us do not know how to get close to Him. We have the illusion that He is so far away and so very unknowable. But He is not. Within you right now, there is a hidden journey taking place. It is an unfolding journey of your *Miraculous Identity.*

What is my miraculous identity? you ask. Your true, miraculous identity is to see yourself as God sees you. It is to experience all He says about who you are, why he created you, realizing your life purpose, and experiencing who God is for you. He designed you to be in relationship with Him and live your life in all of the miraculous wonders He promised you.

This book meets you where you are right now in your *hidden journey.* Opening these pages is rather like floating down a river of living water—sometimes you drift slowly and other times you experience the exhilaration of rushing waters! Revelation of your personal, one-on-one relationship with God will become clearer. He knows you. And He knows how to engage with you.

HOW TO GO THROUGH THIS BOOK

This ten-chapter book will give you a renewing-your-mind upgrade in your *Miraculous Identity.* In Christ, your miraculous identity already exists, you are simply coming into agreement with it. It is interactive and on your part—proactive, providing you with tools to wrap your mind and heart and mind around. Each chapter contains:

- Teaching Section
- Posturing Declarations
- Experiential Activations
- Prayer Focus
- Heavenly Word

Teaching

Each teaching section will bring understanding to a facet of your identity and will likely stir your emotions to have an increased desire for a deeper relationship with God. You are designed to feel God in your emotions. He gave you emotions so you could feel things. You are supposed to experience God with your emotions. The fruit of the Spirit is love, joy, peace, patience, kindness, goodness, faithfulness, and self-control—all involving your emotions.

[handwritten note in margin: fruits only 8 left out gentleness]

God designed you to not just know that He loves you but to *experience* His love. Yes! *Experience* His love in your relationship with Him! He created you to feel His love so much that your response is to believe Him and trust Him and desire Him. You are His beloved.

The Teaching Section prepares you to move right into the Posturing Declarations.

Posturing Declarations

The Posturing Declarations are personalized verses from the Old and New Testaments written in first person for you to speak every day for seven days. You have a proactive role to rewire your thinking about God. This is something only *you* can do. Each chapter will help you create a new habit of renewing your mind. When you renew your mind, a miraculous transformation takes place. Your part is to renew your mind; God does the transformation inside of you. Romans 12:2 Passion Translation reads:

Stop imitating the ideals and opinions of the culture around you, but be inwardly transformed by the Holy Spirit through a total reformation of How you think. This will empower you to discern God's will as you live a beautiful life, satisfying and perfect in his eyes.

Since you will speak the declarations twice a day for one week, I suggest you take one week for each chapter. You don't have to. This course is for you to absorb any way you want. It is not an opportunity to beat yourself up if you don't get everything done. I encourage you to engage with the Posturing Declarations and the additional activations to glean the greatest benefit from this book. If you do nothing else, speak the declarations. Declarations are the heart of this course. Incredible transformation takes place if you *do* the course and not just *read* the course.

Experiential Activations

Activations are interactive and will involve all your senses. They will help you personally engage with the identity target for each chapter. So, take your time and enjoy the process. Each activation section begins with a guide and tracking system for doing the Posturing Declarations. Continue over the week to do the rest of the activations.

Prayer Focus and Heavenly Word

The Prayer Focus is just a starting place for you, a launching pad. Add your own words. The Heavenly Word reflects God's view of your miraculous identity.

The Full Course

The full course can be used as for Bible Study groups, ministry schools, entire church study, and individual study. It includes this book, a workbook, and a video set. The workbook asks questions about the teaching and gives you a place to do your work. The video set includes eleven videos of the author that complement each chapter. It is not the identical teaching as the book; it adds to the teaching.

You are now ready to begin the hidden journey of your miraculous identity. I pray wondrous, wild, exhilarating encounters and revelations upon you. I pray fresh insights and closeness. I pray you experience God's love. And I pray much laughter.

*"Move your heart closer and closer to God,
and he will come even closer to you."*

JAMES 4:8 PASSION TRANSLATION

1

Intimacy with the Nature of God
Just Be Real

Intimate: Very familiar; known very well;
closely acquainted; very personal; most private.

"It's time to say goodbye. My life has been so much better because of you. Our whole marriage has been great because of you. Quacker, I love you." I stood a few more minutes at his bedside while he then told my sister how much she meant to him as well. A bit later, I walked around our backyard to process what had just taken place. Ready or not, like it or not, I faced an unknown future alone. My husband and I had just said our last goodbyes.

I rushed back to his bedside in the living room, sobbing. "I'm sorry you have to see me this way," I said.

His gaze was steady. Surreal. Looking deep into my soul, he said, "*Be real.*"

We had gone to each other countless times for advice over the thirty-plus years we were married. His final piece of wisdom is my most valued treasure.

I asked, "Did I do everything right? You didn't want to be in the hospital, right? You wanted to be at home, right?" He said yes.

He died that night.

His final counsel to me was as gold: *Be real.*

There are times in life when we come to the end of ourselves. With nowhere to go, nowhere to turn, we feel a kind of stirring deep inside, and somehow we know that getting closer to God is the only way to find the next real place. In the face of my pain, I had to have the "real." My hidden journey demanded closeness with God. That's when the vision came. I saw where He was bringing me—to the broad place. The broad place would be like nothing I had ever known. God and only God could take me there. He was the door. I could feel a newness of intimacy with the nature of God.

> *"His love broke open the way and he brought me into a beautiful broad place. He rescued me—because his delight is in me"* (Ps. 18:19 Passion Translation).

God has invited every one of us to come into His presence with confidence and *encounter* Him—our all-knowing, all-seeing, ever-present, miraculous God. Knowing God more intimately develops your understanding and awareness of your miraculous identity. The miraculous God connects with the miraculous you. He pulls on the miraculous you and leads you into a miraculous life with Him. Knowing Him more intimately automatically pulls you into the realm of signs, wonders, and miracles—because those are things He does, and you are His partner. Whether you are a relatively new believer or a very seasoned believer—there is always more, always deeper intimacy with God. God's miraculous world is without limit!

After I said "Yes" to a relationship with God, I wasn't sure exactly *how* to grow closer to Him. I read a book on how to pray an hour a day. The book gave me a strategy and got me started, but I desired a friendship with God to flow between us more naturally. Something fluid and organic—like how two honest-to-goodness best friends enjoy each other. I began setting aside time to pour out my heart to Him and just be with Him. I arose in the middle of the night, when my mind was most quiet. It was perfect for me—no distractions. In the still of the night, I expressed my most intimate thoughts. As my relationship with God the Father began to deepen and grow, and intimacy developed between us, I learned that He also wanted to be with *me*. He *wanted* to spend time with me—He *enjoyed* me. He *loved* me.

> *"I lie awake each night thinking of you and reflecting on how you help me like a father. I sing through the night under your splendor-shadow, offering up to you my songs of delight and joy! With passion I pursue and cling to you. Because I feel your grip on my life, I keep my soul close to your heart"* (Ps. 63:6-8 Passion Translation).

As I share about how my relationship with God grew and developed, I must stress that once you invite Jesus to be Lord of your life, there is no formula for how to draw closer to God. It is a real relationship. You have your own, special, personal relationship with God and your own Spirit-led way of knowing Him more intimately. The main key is to find times to steal away, get alone, and give Him all your attention.

I find times and places where I can be alone and free from distractions. With heavenly boldness, confidence, and humility (Heb. 4:16), I respond to His ever-present invitation to be with Him. Turning all my attention toward God, my heart cries, *"I want more of You, Lord. I want to know You more. I want to go deeper into Your presence."*

At times, God's presence overwhelms me in this place. When His tangible presence encompasses me, I barely want to move a muscle. I might be kneeling, sitting, or lying down; the room feels thick with His presence. With my hands lifted up, I continue to press in further. My heart and mind become postured toward God. Every fiber of my being bows before Him, focusing on Him. I am captivated by His presence. Deep inside I feel a pulling; I sense Him drawing near to me as I draw near to Him. My spirit yearns for more, more of God, more of His presence and intimacy. I am aware of an inward rumbling inside my belly, where rivers of living water are churning and stirring. His Spirit is calling me deeper, to where my innermost being is profoundly connected with His unfathomable depths. I have arrived at that intimate place where *"deep calls unto deep...."* (Psalm 42:7).

> *"Here I am! I stand at the door and knock. If ANYONE hears My voice and opens the door, I will come in and eat with that person, and they with Me"* (Revelation 3:20 NIV).
>
> *"You will seek Me and find Me when you seek Me with all of your heart"* (Jeremiah 29:13 NIV).

Intimacy with God is available for every believer, including YOU. He said it Himself,

God is calling us to intimate friendship with Him.

Powerfully significant, supernatural change happens when we reach this watershed moment. We know we cannot continue on with life as usual when everything within us screams, *"I need more of You, God. I want to really know You."* If you want more of Him in your life, ask Him for greater intimacy and then make room for Him. Give to Him that very thing upon which we place supreme value: Give Him your *time*. The truth is, when you take time to draw near to Him, He draws near to you. I want you to know—this is for YOU.

There's another point I want to make clear: Although feeling His closeness is wonderful, sometimes I don't seem to feel much of anything. When I feel nothing, it doesn't mean He has left me or that something is wrong with me. These seasons happen to all of us. We experience His presence in tangible ways, and sometimes we are there by faith. Walking with the Lord is characterized by faith, not just by feeling or sight. The main thing is to draw near to God.

You don't have to try to be anything or do anything special. You have access to Him 24/7. Simply confide in Him just as you would a close friend. You tell Him secrets, and He tells you secrets. That's what close friends do. They share the intimate secrets of their hearts (Prov. 3:32). You don't have to be a Bible scholar or seminary graduate. You don't have to be a pastor, an elder, a prophet, or Mother Teresa. Just be you.

The next section is a high-level activation where you will purposefully take a position, a posture as a beloved son or daughter of the Most High and speak intimate words to God. We proactively renew our minds. It is not something we pray and ask God to do for us. We do it with intention.

This is your personal time with the One who created you. Speaking love-words of who you really are and who God really is, enter into His presence. These verses are powerful. Find a private place where you won't be disturbed. Tenderly speak these declarations with a quiet, seeking heart.

POSTURING DECLARATIONS

INTIMACY WITH THE NATURE OF GOD

Oh, God, You are my God. Earnestly, I seek you. (Ps. 63:1, 2)

My soul yearns for Your presence. My heart and my flesh cry out for You! (Ps. 84: 2)

My soul thirsts for You, my body longs for You, in a dry and weary land where there is no water. (Ps. 63:1)

I have seen You in the sanctuary and beheld Your power and Your glory. (Ps. 63:1, 2)

Reveal Yourself to me, Lord. Reveal Yourself. (Ps. 63:1, 2)

I love to be in Your presence, Lord. Better is one day in Your courts than a thousand elsewhere! (Ps. 84:10)

On my bed I remember You; I think of You through the watches of the night. (Ps. 63:6)

Whom have I in heaven but You? And being with You, I desire nothing on earth! (Ps.73:25)

I long for a heavenly closeness with You. Draw me close! Draw me! And I will run after you! (Song 1: 4)

Your love is better than wine, better than anything the world has to offer! (Song 1:2)

As the deer pants for water, so my soul pants for You, O God. (Ps. 42:1)

I love you, Lord, with all my heart, with all my soul, with all my mind and with all my strength. (Mark 12:30)

I am passionate to know You! (Jn. 17:3)

Show me great and mighty things that without You, I would not otherwise know. (Jer. 33:3)

Show me marvelous and wondrous things I could never figure out on my own. (Jer. 33:3)

I radiate with love for You, Lord. (Song 6:13)

My face glows with love for You! (Song 6:13)

In Your presence, Lord, I meditate on Your unfailing love. (Ps. 48:9)

Great is Your love, reaching to the heavens; Your faithfulness reaches to the skies. (Ps. 57:10)

I love the sound of Your voice ... and I follow it! (Jn. 10:27)

As I draw near to You, You draw near to me. (Ja. 4:8)

I sing in the shadow of Your wings. (Ps. 63:7)

I stay close to You. (Ps. 63:8)

I confidently and boldly enter into Your presence. (Heb. 4:16)

With You I find grace and mercy in times of need. (Heb. 4:16)

You are my hiding place. (Ps. 32:7)

I am still and I know that You are God. (Ps. 46:10)

I meditate on all Your works and consider all Your mighty deeds. (Ps. 77:12)

I meditate on all the wonderful things You've done for me. (Ps. 77:12)

I seek You and You answer me. You deliver me from all my fears. (Ps. 34:4)

I am an extravagant worshiper. (Song 5:10-16)

I worship You in spirit and in truth. (John 4:23)

You give me dreams and visions and Holy Spirit encounters! (Joel 2:28)

I do not live by bread alone, but by every word that proceeds from Your mouth. (Matt. 4:4)

I am saturated with Your love and affections! (Song 4:1-10)

You are ravished by me! My love is delightful to You, Lord! (Song 4:1-10)

I will go where You want me to go! I will do what You want me to do! (Song 4:16)

I am a lovesick Bride! I am faint with love for You! (Song 2:5)

My love for You is like a blazing fire that many waters cannot quench! (Song 8:6, 7)

I know You desire me! I know You pursue me! (Song 7:10)

I know You love to spend time with me. (Song 7:10)

I am Yours! I am my lover's, and my lover is mine! (Song 6:3)

You fill me with joy in Your presence, with eternal pleasures at Your right hand. (Ps. 16:11)

I delight myself in You, Lord, and You give me the desires of my heart. (Ps 37:4)

I am confident that You never leave me or forsake me! (Heb. 13:5)

You have made known to me the path of life. (Ps. 16:11)

You fill me with joy in Your presence! (Ps. 16:11)

Nothing can separate me from Your love. (Rom. 8:39)

I sing of Your love forever! I declare that Your love stands firm forever! (Ps. 89:1, 2)

One thing I ask of You; this is what I seek: that I may dwell in Your house, Lord, all the days of my life. (Ps. 27:4)

I seek You with all my heart. (Ps. 119:10)

POSTURING INSIGHTS

- When you find you have difficulty believing a posturing verse, you most likely have believed a lie. Take notice: This is a place in your mind that needs to be rewired with God's truth. Write down the lie and then, after it, write the truth according to God's Word.

- You can pray, *"God, I'm sorry for believing the lie, and I break the agreement I have made with the lie. Forgive me. Heal the hurt place in my heart where the lie came in. Fill my heart and mind with Your truth as I speak Your Word. In Jesus' name, Amen."*

EXPERIENTIAL ACTIVATIONS

DIVING INTO THE DEEP END

Activation One

This activation is the most important one in the entire study of your *Miraculous Identity*. Personalizing verses enables you to own them so they become part of you. Jesus told the multitudes,

---

"Seek first the kingdom of God and His righteousness, and all these things shall be added to you" (Matt. 6:33).

Immerse yourself in Intimacy with the Nature of God. Let the posturing declarations drop down into your spirit. The Word of God is alive and will come alive inside you. The personalized verses will move from your mind down into your spirit to the place in you where deep calls unto deep.

Speak the verses aloud daily for one week. Tenderly say them aloud two times a day—in the morning and right before bed. After one week, choose ten of the personalized verses to say once a day for at least thirty days. Increased revelation of intimacy with God will start to become a part of you. Renewing your mind is an action you do intentionally, and this week you are purposefully going after intimacy with God. In doing so, you dismantle opposing mental strongholds. You are proclaiming revelation to the atmosphere *around* you and *within* you. You are a warrior. A pursuer. Diligent. Valiant. Dangerous. The dreaded champion. Going deeper. Going further. May a profound hunger stir inside you. Twice a day.

Activation Two

> *"Draw near to God and He will draw near to you"* (James 4:8).

God's love for us is so vast, so deep, and so wide, and He invites us into that love daily. Sometimes it's easy to run into His loving arms and spend time with Him; sometimes it's difficult. As you posture, you may find difficulty fully believing you can have a close, personal relationship with God. You may be thinking that you don't pray enough or that you don't know the Bible enough. You may think that with the things you've done and the mistakes you've made, this kind of closeness with God isn't available to you. You may think you are not worthy to come into God's presence. There may be a deep place in you where you feel like you are not important. These are lies.

Guess who doesn't want you becoming closer with the God of the universe?

The first step is for your mind to be *renewed*. For this activation, we will focus on a primary verse that counteracts those lies. When anyone draws near to God, God draws near to him. No one is excluded.

Write this verse on paper or post-its and place it above your bathroom mirror on your refrigerator, on your car dashboard, and anywhere else you frequent. When you see it, decree it.

Ask God to forgive you for believing that you could not have a close friendship with Him. Verbally break the agreement you have had with the lie. Say:

Lord, I am sorry for believing I could not get close to You. Forgive me for judging myself so harshly. This lie has kept me from drawing near to you and believing that You draw near to me. All that changes NOW! In Jesus' Name, I break my agreement with that lie. I say that bondage is broken! Lord, heal the injured place in my heart when the lie came in. From now on, I know that when I draw near to You, You draw near to me! I want to get as close to You as I can. And after that—even closer!

Activation Three

Find a private place you can go and spend time with God. It can be a corner of your backyard, the car, or a walk-in closet. Bring paper and a Bible. Wait before Him and listen. Ask Him to tell you what is on His heart. You tell Him what is on your heart. Listen and write down what you are sensing. If you are not feeling much, it's okay. Continue to practice being in His presence. If you lack a strong desire to know Him and spend time with Him, simply ask for that desire.

Activation Four

Play music that really gets you into the Lord's presence and sit completely still, with your eyes closed, focusing everything within you on Him alone. Then, turn off the music to be even more fully engaged with Him. This way, you will not follow the words or the beat of the music. You are still before Him. Ask Him to reveal Himself to you. Ask Him to show you how He sees you. Ask anything about your life. Ask anything about anything. Being intimate means you are seeing into one another.

While you're spending time with God, draw what you feel He is showing you. I love doing this. I get out crayons and colored felt-tipped pens and draw like a third-grader, and I know He loves it. (There will be space in the workbook for this.) What other creative things could you do with God?

PRAYER FOCUS

INTIMACY

Lord, I desire that deeper place of intimacy with You. I am alive with passion for You. I want to know You more. I desire to understand the wonders of Your very nature and become continually transformed into Your likeness. I pursue You with all my heart.
Amen.

HEAVENLY WORD

Beloved, You will seek Me and find me when you seek Me with all your heart. I love being pursued by you. How beautiful you are to Me. You have stolen My heart, My bride, with one glance of your eyes! How delightful is your love, my bride! Let me hear your voice!

JEREMIAH 29:13;

SONG OF SONGS 5:6; 4:1, 9, 10; 8:13

"He who dwells in the secret place of the Most High

shall abide under the shadow of the Almighty."

PSALM 91:1

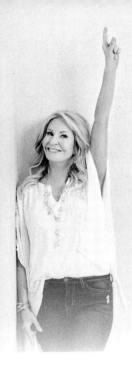

2

The Secret Place
Meeting with God

Secret Place: To hide or be concealed; kept close

The secret place of the Most High is not of this world. It is found in God's world, in the heavenly realms. The beauty of the secret place is that it is a safe place, a hidden place, a realm in the spirit, where you find refuge, safely tucked away from this world's strife. It is a place where you can hear heaven's songs and enjoy sweet fellowship with God. It is here that you find rest for your soul, where your spirit is invigorated, and where your body is renewed. The Most High God has extended to all who are thirsty His invitation to the secret place. The call is to all who hunger for greater closeness with God. *Come! Let anyone who is thirsty come!*

Whenever you steal away to be quiet with God, you can enter the secret place. In the secret place of the Most High, you are a warrior, and you are a lover—a lover who passionately loves Jesus, always desiring more of Him. You also are a warrior who aggressively pursues God and His prophetic promises. The combination of lover/warrior makes you wild and unpredictable in the world's eyes because you desire to do only what you see your Father doing. You aren't led by circumstance or swayed by man. You walk to heaven's rhythm.

When you spend time with God, you become more and more like Him. In His presence you are transformed. It is much like picking up the attributes of a good friend you frequently spend time with. Just like you begin to speak with the same phrases as your friend and begin to think like your friend, so you begin to take on God's character when you spend time with Him and get to know Him. As you saturate yourself with His presence, yokes of bondage break off and invisible prisons that held you captive are weakened and dissolved, floating away downstream. You are cleansed and refreshed in the secret place of the Most High. He exchanges His yoke—a yoke that is light and easy to bear—for your burdensome one.

As you are healed and refreshed, it is natural to become filled with His passions. A desire grows to learn what is on your Father's heart. In the secret place your love for people grows and your capacity for love enlarges. He enables you to love from a selfless place where your heart motives become ever purer. You love the Bride, and you love the unlovely. All because of Him.

Yet, in the secret place even more heavenly treasures reside. After all your thanksgiving and praise and worship. After all your petitions and prayers. Even after speaking to Him in a heavenly language and inner groans of the Spirit, if you keep pressing in and are willing to be quiet, you enter into a deep, still communion with Him. It is the *"Be still and know I am God"* place. The word "know" does not mean intellectual knowledge—it means experiential knowledge. You are one with Him—where you are in Him and He is in you. Revelation is present when you are deep in the secret place of the Most High. If you can just *be* with Him in stillness, He reveals so much. Here, He shows you great and unsearchable things you would not otherwise know. If you long for greater revelation, posture for going deep into the secret place.

Miraculous Identity is not a "how to" book. It is not even a self-help book. *Miraculous Identity* is a book designed to stir a hunger in you to not only comprehend how miraculous your identity really is but also to catapult you into deeper intimacy with God. I suspect something is happening to you already, because it is happening to me as I write. Just talking about knowing Him more intimately stirs a greater desire inside me to steal away and be alone with Him.

The next section is a high-level activation where you will purposefully take a position, a posture as a beloved son or daughter of the Most High and speak intimate words of dwelling in the secret place. We proactively renew our minds. It is not something we pray and ask God to do for us. We do it with intention. With love-words flowing from your mouth about who you really are and who God is, enter the Lord's presence These verses are powerful. Find a private place where you won't be disturbed. Tenderly speak these decrees with a quiet, seeking heart.

POSTURING DECLARATIONS

THE SECRET PLACE

I dwell in the secret place of the Most High. (Ps. 91:1)

I abide under the shadow of the Almighty! (Ps. 91:1)

You are my refuge and my fortress; My God, in You I will trust." (Ps. 91:1)

You cover me with Your feathers, and under Your wings, I find refuge. (Ps. 91:4)

Your faithfulness is my shield and rampart. (Ps. 91:4)

In the day of trouble, You conceal me in Your tabernacle. In the secret place of Your tent You hide me. You lift me up on a rock. (Ps. 27:5)

You hide me in the secret place of Your presence from the conspiracies of man. (Ps. 31:20)

I am so safe with You. You are my place of safety. (Ps. 18:2)

I am still. I know You are God. (Ps. 46:10)

I calm and quiet my soul. (Ps. 131:2)

The work of righteousness is peace, and the effect will be quietness and confidence forever. (Isa. 32:17)

In quietness and trust is my strength. (Isa. 30:15)

I am still before You and wait patiently for You. (Ps. 37:7)

The Lord is in His holy temple. Let all the earth be silent before Him. (Hab. 2:20)

I am seated with Jesus in heavenly places. I see things and know things from this high place I could not otherwise know. You are the Revealer. (Eph. 2:6)

I have spiritual food to eat people know nothing about. (Jn. 4:32)

I come into Your garden. And partake of the sweet fragrances ... eat the honeycomb ... drink the milk and wine. I drink deeply of Your love! (Song 5:1)

You are my hiding place. (Ps. 32:7)

You preserve me from trouble. (Ps. 32:7)

You surround me with songs of deliverance. (Ps. 32:7)

You are a defense for the helpless, a refuge from the storm, a shade from the heat. You are everything to me. (Ps. 25:4)

You surround me with songs of deliverance. (Ps. 32:7)

With You, I find rest for my soul. Such sweet rest! (Matt. 11:28)

When I am thirsty, I come to You. I drink, and I'm fulfilled. (Jn. 7:37)

The angel of the Lord encamps around me, and He delivers me! (Ps. 34:7)

I find refuge in the Lord. His faithfulness is my shield and rampart. (Ps. 91:4)

I am kept and protected from the evil one. (Jn. 17:15)

I am hidden with Christ in God. (Col. 3:3)

As the mountains surround Jerusalem, so the Lord surrounds me both now and forevermore. (Ps. 125:2)

In God, whose word I praise, in God I trust; I will not be afraid. What can mortal man do to me? (Ps. 56:4)

Some trust in chariots and some in horses, but I trust in the name of the Lord my God. (Ps. 20:7)

I enter into the Lord's rest. (Matt. 11:28)

Jesus is my peace. (Eph. 2:14)

I go out with joy and am led forth with peace. You watch over me and take care of me no matter where I am. (Isa. 55:12)

I am in perfect peace because my mind is focused on the You. I trust You. (Isa. 26:3)

I cast my cares on You, and You sustain me. You never let the righteous fall. (Ps. 55:22)

I cast all my cares on You because You care for me! (1 Pet. 5:7)

You are my refuge and strength and an ever-present help in times of trouble. (Ps. 46:1)

You keep my lamp burning. You turn my darkness into light. (Ps. 18:28)

I see visions and dream dreams. I know secret things given to me by You. (Joel 2:28)

I have set You, Lord, always before me. Because You are at my right hand, I will not be shaken. (Ps. 16:8)

I do not fear the terror of night, nor the arrow that flies by day, not the pestilence that stalks in the darkness, not the plague that destroys at midday. (Ps. 91:5, 6)

A thousand may fall at my side, ten thousand at my right hand, but it will not come near me! (Ps. 91:7)

I am hidden in the shadow of Your wings. (Ps. 17:8)

I am hidden in the secret place. The secret place where I meet with You. Safe and set apart with You. In the Secret Place. (Ps. 31:20)

POSTURING INSIGHTS

- When you find you have difficulty believing a posturing verse, you most likely have believed a lie. Take notice: This is a place in your mind that needs to be rewired with God's truth. Write down the lie and then, after it, write the truth according to God's Word.

- You can pray, *"God, I'm sorry for believing the lie, and I break the agreement I have made with the lie. Forgive me. Heal the hurt place in my heart where the lie came in. Fill my heart and mind with Your truth as I speak Your Word. In Jesus' name, Amen."*

EXPERIENTIAL ACTIVATIONS

ENTERING THE SECRET PLACE

Activation One

That you are reading this book indicates your desire for more than a superficial relationship with God. You want more. The desire inside you causes you to become militant and to aggressively pursue God. Miraculous identity means being miraculously close to God, and through deep relationship with Him you enter the secret place.

Read the personalized verses twice a day—first thing in the morning and right before bed. Then, after one week, choose ten verses to continue to proclaim for the next thirty days. This is not a religious exercise. You are proactively renewing your mind. This requires discipline. And, yes, sometimes, you may not feel like doing it. Do it anyway. Develop perseverance. Give your passion and strength to seeking Him (Heb. 11:6). Write out the personalized verses or start a posturing file on your computer and rotate the ten verses.

I encourage you. You've got this. You are developing a habit, a lifestyle.

> *"We throw open our doors to God and discover at the same moment he has already thrown open his door to us We find ourselves standing where we always hoped we might stand— out in the wide-open spaces of God's grace and glory, standing tall and shouting our praise"* (Romans 5:2 Message).

Activation Two

We open the door and find He is already there! God is relentless. He continually draws you into His secret place, the secret place of His presence. You long to go there with Him, but maybe you've had a hard time drawing close when you postured in the verses. If any of the verses were difficult for you to believe, choose a few of them and write them down.

Then, ask God to show you why you had a hard time believing them. When we have a hard time believing God, we have undoubtedly believed a lie—something in opposition to what God has said. Remember how the serpent got Eve to question God and believe a lie? The serpent said to Eve, *"Did God really say…?"* (Gen. 3:1).

Ask God to show you the lie you have adopted in place of the truth of the verse. Once you see the lie, quiet your heart and ask God to forgive you for believing the lie. Next, verbally break the agreement you have had with the lie. Say: *"Lord, I am sorry for believing the lie. It kept me from believing Your Word. In Jesus' name, I break my agreement with that lie. The bondage is broken! From now on, I believe."* Say the verse again in your own words.

Now take some to time let God heal any place in your heart was affected by the lie. Say, *"Lord, heal the injured place in my heart when the lie came in. I…"*

Be real. Be transparent. Know that He draws you close as He heals your heart. God is continually interacting with you. He draws you, gives you revelation, and transforms you—continually. As you go through *Miraculous You*, more and more you will recognize how God is always engaged with you. And your sensitivity to the Spirit of God will expand. That is where we will go in the next chapter. It is going to be awesome!

Activation Three

Activation three is a very experiential activation for entering in and being in the secret place of the Most High. The secret place can be a physical location you go to meet with god, but it most often connotes a state of your soul in relationship with God. We meet with Him in the secret places of the heart. Here, we commune with Him— transparently and honestly. Matthew 6:6 offers a great description:

> *"When you pray, go into your room, and when you have shut your door, pray to your Father who is in the secret place; and your Father who sees in secret will reward you openly."*

After posturing in the secret place verses, think about your secret place as being within you. Close your eyes, and focus on a place deep within your core. Posture in that inner place and spend time with God. Keep it simple. Just be quiet and relax there. Relax your whole self in this place of solitude with Him. Watch and see if you can feel His presence there.

If you have the workbook, you can write about your time with Him.

Activation Four

When you are in the secret place, you posture yourself from where you are truly seated—where God raised you up with Christ and seated you with Him in the heavenly realms far above all rule and authority, power and dominion, and every negative manifestation (Eph. 1:20-23; 2:6). Wow! Yep, that's you.

Think of a circumstance that is trying to stir up a storm in your life. Declare to it that you are seated in heavenly realms with Christ Jesus. Really ponder this truth.

Rewrite these verses from Ephesians in your own words. Speak to your challenging situation using words from these verses. These verses reflect the secret place. Pull them in close to the inner secret place in your belly. From out of your belly—which is the same as your innermost being—is the place from which rivers of living waters flow! Now think about that. Close your eyes and sense the rivers of living waters (John 7:38). Look up that verse, then close your eyes and focus on this truth. Really ponder it. Listen to me. Don't hurry back to your life. This is your time. Give God that which is a most valuable commodity: your time.

Activation Five

The dictionary defines *refuge* as *a condition of being safe or sheltered from pursuit, danger, or trouble.* If you look it up in Strong's Concordance #4268, you will see it defined as a shelter (literally or figuratively)—hope, place of refuge, shelter, and trust. In a child-like way, draw a picture of the secret place—your place of refuge.

What are the colors? Are there sounds? Is there fragrance? Atmosphere?

You will find a place in the workbook to create your inner image on paper. Be as a child and draw outside the lines. In other words: don't think you have to create perfect work of art. Draw from your heart. God loves this about you! He loves the expressions of your heart.

PRAYER FOCUS

ENTERING THE SECRET PLACE

Dear Lord, I choose to enter Your presence. Hide me in the secret place of Your presence. Take hold of my hand and pull me into You. Take me to the secret place where I can rest in Your shadow. Show me Your abiding place. Teach me

how to eat spiritual food and drink from Your wellspring. Enable me to feel Your presence. I open my spiritual senses! I open eyes and ears so that I fully enjoy You. I open my ears to hear heavenly sounds and my sense of smell so I can discern heavenly fragrances. I open my entire being to the secret place of an intimate, glorious friendship with You!
Amen

HEAVENLY WORD

Dear Precious One, I am your shelter. Abide in My shadow. Hide yourself in My Word. When you do so, you will be like a tree planted along the riverbank, bearing fruit each season. I am your refuge—your trustworthy place. I know you become weary and burdened. Come to Me. Dive into the secret place of the Most High, and I will give you rest. I will restore your soul. In the secret place, I will pour into you all that you need. My yoke is easy and My burden is light.

PSALM 91:1-2; PSALM 1:2-3;
MATTHEW 11:28-30

"The wind blows wherever it pleases. You hear its sound, but you cannot tell where it comes from or where it is going. So it is with everyone born of the Spirit."

JOHN 3:8

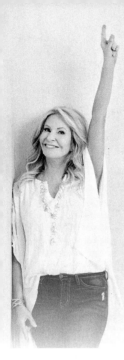

3

The Wind of the Spirit
Inside You

Wind: Spirit, breath, wind

"He is like the wind. When the wind blows, you can't control it. You want to control the conversation, but Holy Spirit is interrupting it." My mentor nailed it. I thought I had waited patiently during the two cell phone calls he took—but I hadn't. And he saw I was annoyed. "The Holy Spirit is always doing something, Linda, and you can't control it," he said. "He's like the *wind*. You think those calls were interruptions, but both calls were from people who had come up in our conversation. That's Holy Spirit confirming what I was saying. Do you see that?" I had to admit that until my dear friend called my attention to it, I did not. How easily I lost awareness of the ever-present involvement of Holy Spirit in my life.

Jesus said He would be going away, but would not leave us all alone. He would send us *another* Helper (John 14:15-18). The word "another" is significant. It literally means another of the same kind—meaning this helper would be just like Jesus. In other words, you have someone just like Jesus walking around with you all the time.

Holy Spirit is a Person. He's the third Person of the Trinity. He is as much God as Jesus and God the Father. But let me ask a few important questions: Are you conscious of Him? Are you engaged in conversation with Him? Are you developing a relationship with Him? Do you sense the wind of the Spirit moving you and directing you?

Like an untethered boat driven by the wind, we are carried by the wind of the Spirit as we yield to Him. He blows us wherever He wants us to go. We are on the adventure of our lives, with Him leading us, moving us, and revealing heavenly secrets to us. Even during what we think are insignificant moments—like phone interruptions during a conversation—the Holy Spirit is constantly revealing insights and confirming our future. Even right now, as you are absorbing this passage, He is working with you. The Holy Spirit is the Spirit of Truth, and He leads us unto *all truth*. He is the great Revealer, continually revealing secrets to us—things only God knows. Life with Holy Spirit is far more exciting than any Disneyland ride or bungee jump. Life with Him is unpredictable and enormously supernatural.

Once you choose Jesus as Lord of your life, a relationship with Holy Spirit begins. Is it possible to be about your business without any awareness of Him? Yes. But it doesn't have to be that way. The Holy Spirit is in the middle of everything. When you are asking, *"Where is God in the middle of this mess I'm in?"* He is right there. He is your Helper, and He helps you with everything. Just like the Bible says, He never leaves you nor forsakes you. Plus, if you're not supposed to do something, He'll let you know as you increase your awareness of Him.

The Book of Acts provides an insider-look as to what life is like *with* Holy Spirit. As a young believer, I marked every reference to Holy Spirit in Acts. I learned so much about this marvelous Person Jesus sent to be my Guide. The early church was immersed in day-to-day fellowship with Holy Spirit. They relied on Him for everything. At one point, they even said how an idea *"...seemed good to Holy Spirit and to us..."* (Acts 15:28).

No wonder! In Acts 1:8, Jesus told His disciples, *"You will receive power when the Holy Spirit comes on you…"*

We are not to be ruled by externals. Following externals—circumstances and our own ideas about how we can make our futures work out—causes us to be subject to that realm. It produces fear and anxiety. The Holy Spirit's plan does not include this kind of stress. Our spiritual DNA aches to be led by the Holy Spirit, as Jesus was (Matthew 4:1). He wasn't led by circumstance or even need. The Holy Spirit always directed Him. What he saw the Father doing, He did. What He heard the Father saying, He said. As our relationship with the Holy Spirit develops, we must be still … and listen. In those still moments, we learn to follow Him. Our outward walk is directed from a deep inward place. As we grow, we can be in a war zone with bombs going off and be able to hear and follow His lead. Yes, it takes time and focus to be postured like this, but this is exactly where you are headed. And what a sweet place it is!

Wouldn't you know it, as I write today a strong wind is blowing outside my window. I see the powerful effects of the wind—leaves, branches, and entire trees swaying. I hear the mighty wind whipping through the trees and around the house. If I stepped outside, my hair would blow in twenty directions. Where the wind is coming from, I can only guess. Where it is going, I do not know. It leaves nearly everything in motion: Flowering vines dancing, pool water rippling, pillows flying off patio furniture. I could position myself to resist the Holy Spirit like a giant boulder resists the wind. What does the Bible call it? Stubborn and stiff-necked (Acts 17:51). Or I could yield to the wind like a reed bowing low, humbling and submitting.

The Bible speaks of wind, breath, and Spirit about the Holy Spirit. What if the wind were blowing *inside* my house? I'd see papers flying, vases falling over, chandeliers swinging sideways. What if this wind blew inside *me*? What would that feel like? Would everything in me fall into alignment with His purposes? Would He blow out all the unhealed places? Would He breathe life into my dreams and visions?

Would I be filled with the breath of heaven? You bet. Close your eyes and pause right now. Focus on the wind of the Spirit within you. Can you feel that? Just reading those words about the inner reality of the Spirit causes me to be more in tune with His presence.

God has given you a miraculous identity totally separate from this natural world. You are called into a miraculous, supernatural life of signs and wonders and relationship. Right now, you walk in so much engagement with the Spirit of God in your everyday life that most of the time, you *do not* even recognize it! Why? Because the miraculous presence of God flows so *naturally* through you as you lean into Him. Think about it: Experiencing joy when tribulation invades your life is *miraculous*. Being thankful in times of deep distress is *miraculous*. Opening your heart and feeling God's love when you see yourself as inadequate, insecure, and with low self-esteem is *miraculous*. God's miraculous power flowing through you yields responses and inner reactions that are contrary to this world. You live in the world yet function in your miraculous identity all at the same time simultaneously!

As you posture today, verse after verse will pour out from your mouth, unveiling the Person of the Holy Spirit. Just like the rest of the Bible, these verses are alive. With increased understanding, your relationship with the Holy Spirit will blossom. I pray the breath of God upon this posturing day for you. I pray great revelation and transformational encounters as you drink in more of the Spirit of the Living God! Right now, speak these personalized verses about Holy Spirit and you.

POSTURING DECLARATIONS

HOLY SPIRIT, I WANT TO KNOW YOU!

Jesus, You did not leave me all alone. (Jn. 14:16)

You sent the Holy Spirit to be with me forever! (Jn. 14:16)

Holy Spirit, You are with me and in me. (Jn. 14:16)

You are with me all the time. Right now, You are not only at my side, but you also live in me. (Jn. 14:16, 17)

You are the Spirit of Truth! (Jn. 16:13)

You are always revealing Truth to me! (Jn. 16:13)

Right now, You're breathing on me. (Jn. 16:13)

Right now, You're breathing in me. (Jn. 16:13)

Right now, You're breathing through me. (Jn. 16:13)

Wonderful Holy Spirit, You teach me. (Jn. 14:26)

You are the Revealer. (Jn. 16:13)

Reveal to me deep things of God. (1 Cor. 2:10)

Reveal hidden mysteries. (Jn. 16:15)

You are my Helper, called to my side as an intercessor. (Jn. 15:26)

A Comforter. (Jn. 15:26)

A Counselor. (Jn. 15:26)

You give me great ideas! (Jn. 15:26)

And You partner with me on those ideas. (Jn. 15:26)

Holy Spirit, I eagerly desire the gifts You have for me! (1 Cor. 14:1)

Holy Spirit, I drink You in. (Jn. 7:37)

Holy Spirit, I breathe You in. (Jn. 7:37)

Drinking from the fountain of Your Spirit, I am refreshed and sustained. (1 Cor. 12:13)

From my innermost being flows rivers of living water—rivers of the Spirit. (Jn. 7:38)

No one knows the things of God except the Spirit of God. (1 Cor. 2:11)

I have received the Spirit who is from God so I may know what God has freely given me. (1 Cor. 2:12)

I am postured like Apostle Paul—my message is not with enticing words of man's wisdom, but with a demonstration of the Spirit and of power! (1 Cor. 2:4-5)

Confirm Your Word with signs following it.
(Mk.16:20)

I have my mind set on what the Holy Spirit
desires. (Rom. 8:5)

I seek those things that gratify the Holy Spirit.
(Rom. 8:5)

I am not following externals; I am living the life
of the Spirit. (Rom. 8:9)

I deeply desire You to orchestrate my day. So,
orchestrate my day, Holy Spirit! (Rom. 8:9)

I often do not know what to pray but, Holy
Spirit, YOU do! Intercede for me with groans
that words cannot express! (Rom. 8:26)

I put up my sail and allow myself to be driven
along by the wind of the Spirit. (Acts 27:15)

I am moved by the wind of the Spirit! (Jn. 3:8)

I am led by the wind of the Spirit! (Jn. 3:8)

Wind of the Spirit, Come! Blow in my home!
(Jn. 3:8)

Come! Blow in my life! (Jn. 3:8)

Come! Mighty Wind of the Spirit, blow within
me! (Jn. 3:8)

POSTURING INSIGHTS

- When you find you have difficulty believing a posturing verse, you most likely have believed a lie. Take notice: This is a place in your mind that needs to be rewired with God's truth. Write down the lie and then, after it, write the truth according to God's Word.

- You can pray, *"God, I'm sorry for believing the lie, and I break the agreement I have made with the lie. Forgive me. Heal the hurt place in my heart where the lie came in. Fill my heart and mind with Your truth as I speak Your Word. In Jesus' name, Amen."*

EXPERIENTIAL ACTIVATIONS

YIELDING TO THE WIND OF THE SPIRIT

Activation One

Posturing in *Holy Spirit, I Want to Know You!* will plant key verses about the Holy Spirit in your heart, enabling an increased awareness of His presence. Understanding the nature of Holy Spirit, what He does, and how He functions as part of the Trinity affects your ability to recognize the many ways He relates to you throughout the day.

Personal note: I'm so used to Him being referred to as "the" Holy Spirit that I do this often myself. But then, because He is a person, I will also refer to Him directly as Holy Spirit. I use these ways of addressing Him interchangeably.

For this activation, your assignment is to proclaim these verses for one week—first thing in the morning when you get up and right before you go to bed. After one week of posturing twice a day, choose ten verses to speak once a day for thirty days. Continuing this lifestyle of proclaiming God's Word allows the truths to continue to renew your mind, drop down into your spirit and ultimately become a vibrant facet of your miraculous identity.

When I became a Christian, I wanted to learn everything I could about Holy Spirit. I came out of the new age movement and, after so much deception, I fervently wanted to know the Spirit of Truth. Since the book of Acts reveals the power of the Spirit in the early church (Acts 1:8), I read through Acts and marked every time the Holy Spirit is mentioned or when His power is demonstrated.

This is the second part of activation one: Read through Acts and note every time there is a demonstration of the Holy Spirit. Your eyes will be opened to how intimately early church believers knew Holy Spirit. He was so real to them. Regarding an idea they had, they said, *Holy Spirit and us though it was a good idea* (Acts 15:28).

Activation Two

Fasten your seatbelts, because I am going to share something very important! What I am about to say might sound like it is contrary to the emphasis in this book on proclaiming verses about miraculous identity—but it is not. When you are in the throes of transition and transformation and are going through a very difficult passage, God is right there with you. He is holding you up and sustaining you. It was during extremely difficult seasons of loss, betrayal, and severe anxiety that I learned what I am about to tell you. When you understand this, you enter His rest.

During many transitional seasons of your life, know this: *You can't proclaim your way through it. He carries you through it.*

This passage exemplifies this truth:

> *"Are you tired? Worn out? Burned out on religion? Come to me. Get away with me and you'll recover your life. I'll show you how to take a real rest. Walk with me and work with me—watch how I do it. Learn the unforced rhythms of grace. I won't lay anything heavy or ill-fitting on you. Keep company with me and you'll learn to live freely and lightly"* (Matt. 11:28-30 Message).

As you go through this book, I don't want you to feel that proclaiming verses is a weight on your shoulders. It is not. I command that concept to lift off your shoulders right now, in Jesus' name. Proclaiming verses renews your mind and aligns your thought-life identity with how heaven sees you. You are simply adhering to Romans 12:1-2, and as you do so, God Almighty does the unseen, inner transformative work deep within you.

In this activation, you will practice connecting to the place inside you, where deep calls unto deep and rivers of living waters spring forth. Right now, pray out loud in the Spirit (Jude 1:20) and think about praying in your head. Concentrate on hearing your voice in your head.

After about a minute, pray in the Spirit and focus on your mouth. Think about how the sounds of words are in your mouth.

Now, you will go to the headwaters of the Holy Spirit. Drop your focus down to deep within your belly and pray in the Spirit from there. Keep going. Think about how Jesus said that rivers of living waters will flow from deep within your belly. Stay here for a while. Think about how rivers coming together churn and stir and are vibrant with great force.

Do this activation as part of your prayer time throughout the week. You will have a place in the workbook to write your experience.

Activation Three

The third activation is an outdoor adventure. Go outside and experience the movement of the wind. There may be a gentle breeze or a super strong wind blowing. Most often it is barely a whisper of movement. Ask Holy Spirit to teach you about how He moves by watching the movement of the natural wind. Watch how everything moves in the wind. How does the wind feel on your face? Now focus your attention of the wind moving inside you. What is He doing inside you? Jot down your insights.

Activation Four

During Jesus' final hours before He was arrested and crucified, He taught the disciples about the person of the Holy Spirit. Here are some verses that will tell you more about Holy Spirit:

John 14:15-18, 25-26
John 15:25-27
John 16:12-14
Acts 1;1-2, 1;8
Acts 2

Look them up and write what they reveal about Holy Spirit. If you have the workbook, you will have a place to write your notes.

PRAYER FOCUS

LED BY THE SPIRIT

Holy Spirit, I am becoming more aware of Your presence. You are always with me. You never leave me. I want to be sensitive to You, to see You in action. I am purposefully postured to see beyond my circumstances. I am Your partner, doing all the fun God stuff with You, alongside You—not ahead of You or lagging behind You. I am so hungry to develop a deeper relationship with You. Holy Spirit, fill me!
Amen.

HEAVENLY WORD

Dear One, The wind of My Spirit is always moving you. Even when you don't feel the wind, I am blowing on your heart and directing you and enveloping you. Yield to My Spirit and how you are propelled along. I sent Him to be your best friend, your Revealer, and your Guide. My Spirit is so much fun! Being carried by My Spirit is a blast! You can be going in one direction and suddenly find yourself sailing in another. You go up and around and sideways and do loop-de-loops! Find freedom in Me. Enjoy Me. I enjoy you!

JOHN 3:8; REVELATION 1:10; JOHN 14:26;
ACTS 8:39-40; 2 CORINTHIANS 3:17

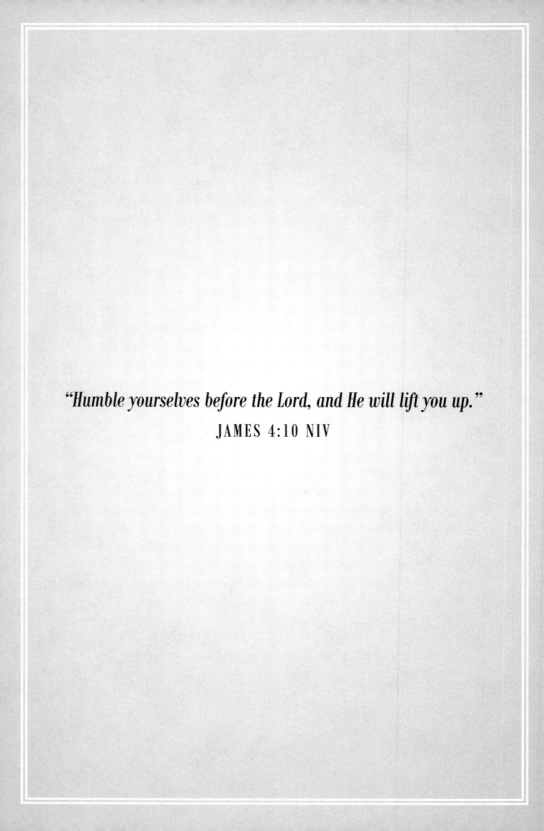

"Humble yourselves before the Lord, and He will lift you up."

JAMES 4:10 NIV

4

Humility
You Don't Have to Make Your Own Way

Humble: to make low … to lower oneself. It describes a person
who is devoid of all arrogance and self-exaltation—a person
who is willingly submitted to God and His will.[1]

I t's not all on your shoulders to make things happen. You do not
have to figure out everything. Just breathe. Let go. You have a
partner. You do not need to force your own way. You can have
passion and drive and vision—and know the God of the universe is
your partner. He opens doors for you. He gives you favor. He will
bring people into your life at the right time. He is always working on
your behalf. He will lift you up. That means He will make your life
significant. Humility is yielding to His lead.

I am not talking about worldly humility. God's view of you and
humility is miraculous. Worldly humility too often means groveling
before others, thinking you are no good, and that everyone else is
better. Biblical humility is stepping away from pride and arrogance.

---

[1]   New Spirit Filled Life Bible, p. 1323

The facet of humility we are going to focus on is what it means to be humble before the Lord.

You have dreams and visions that are way beyond your abilities. You *know* you do not have the resources to see these dreams fulfilled. The truth is, you cannot accomplish anything of eternal significance without Him. Period. Humility before the Lord is recognizing you need God's help.

A couple nights ago, I was feeling anxious about being able to write this book and do it well. Exasperated, I said to Him: *"I don't know enough!"* Before I could take in my next breath, He answered: *"It's okay. I know everything."* In a flash, I was flooded with trust and confidence.

With humility coursing through your veins, pride and arrogance are not part of your identity equation. You know in your knower the Holy Spirit is making the way for you. The next door he has for you doesn't open when you are a long way from it. It opens when you get right in front of it. You must be going in the right direction— toward the door. But we always have a choice to go through it. You depend on God for His help, His direction, His provision. Humility is *knowing* God will raise you up at exactly the right time in His big picture. You move forward, hand in hand with Him. The feel of His hand guides you, and you sense whether you are to move to the left or the right. You flow with Him. Following His lead. What does this look like? Bowing low, before Him.

I'll give an example, a prophetic act that demonstrates humility.

A pastor friend of mine was attending a conference, and when it came time to receive the offering, he pulled out his wallet and asked God what He wanted him to give. The pastor heard God say, "I want you to give Me *you*." The pastor walked down the aisle to the front of the auditorium and stretched out his six-foot-plus frame across the front of the platform. He had long since given God everything he was or ever hoped to be. Yet, at God's request, he humbled himself, not caring what anyone thought and literally acted out what is written in Romans 12:1 (NIV):

> "... to offer your bodies as a living sacrifice, holy and pleasing to God—this is your true and proper worship."

I am not suggesting that you run to the front of your church and sprawl out on the platform. There are a lot of ways to offer your life to God. The point is, when you give Him your life on all accounts, you are humbling yourself before Him. Humility is a posture of the heart and an attitude in the mind. Do you see your life as a living sacrifice to God? Does your heart say, *"I can't do this life thing alone. God, I need You!"* With humility permeating your life, your dreams are compelled to bow low before Him. Everything you say, do, and think are ways of bowing before Him and *acknowledging* Him. This is when, according to Proverbs 3:5-6 (NIV), He directs your path.

> "Trust in the Lord with all your heart and lean not on your own understanding: in all your ways acknowledge him, and he will direct your paths."

A major key: How can He direct what is not submitted?

God *opposes* the proud and shows favor to the humble. Hmm ... hard to digest, isn't it? When we are proud, we get pretty much zippo—at least from God. Here's the same idea from 1 Peter 5:5-6:

> *"In every relationship, each of you must wrap around yourself the apron of a humble servant, Because God resists you when you are proud but multiplies grace and favor when you are humble. If you bow low in God's awesome presence, he will eventually exalt you as you leave the timing in his hands."*

You are the one who chooses the way of humility. The *miraculous identity* inside you draws you like a magnet toward humility. But you are the one who chooses it. You clothe yourself in humility. God's grace, His supernatural ability, flows through us when we choose to posture ourselves bowing low before Him. And then the miraculous occurs: *He lifts us up in perfect timing.*

Do you really want to fulfill everything God has called you to do? You don't have to figure it all out on your own. He already has it figured out. Relax. No stress. No having to be perfect. Go into the secret place. That intimate place. The real. Your hidden journey.

Over the past year, I have ministered with a team in three developing countries, Costa Rica, Columbia, and Dominican Republic. The people in these countries have very little, are very poor, very humble, and passionate for God. Most have few belongings, little education, low-wage job, and no car—basically nothing materially. They know they can't make it on their own. Their childlike faith puts a demand on God for miracles. For every need, every sickness, every threat, they must put absolute trust in God. There is no plan B. God is all they've got. And there, in the poorest of nations, people are healed and delivered. Why? Humility. Humility is another door to your miraculous identity. Humility is demonstrated outwardly from an inner, hidden transformation taking place because of a renewed mind. Humility begins to assume the posture of a servant. We are not here on earth to be served but to serve. Look at Mark 10:42-45 NIV:

> *"Jesus called them together and said, "You know that those who are regarded as rulers of the Gentiles lord it over them, and their high officials exercise authority over them. Not so with you. Instead, whoever wants to become great among you must be your servant, and whoever wants to be first must be slave of all. For even the Son of Man did not come to be served, but to serve, and to give his life as a ransom for many."*

I believe miracles come more easily in these nations than in advanced cultures because the people have become so humble. The key is found in Matthew 5:3. The Amplified Bible reads:

> *"Blessed (happy, to be envied, and spiritually prosperous—with life-joy and satisfaction in God's favor and salvation, regardless of their outward conditions) are the poor in spirit (the humble, who rate themselves insignificant), for theirs is the kingdom of heaven."*

Personally, I don't have a "Plan B." Ahead of all my plans is God. Ahead of all medical options, financial advisors, business plans, relationship plans, ideas, goals—is God.

Just speaking these words for Posturing in Humility won't make you humble. But because of the power of the Word, posturing in humility will help shift your heart to lean toward humility. And speaking the Word will be instrumental in renewing your mind into the posture of humility. You bind yourself to words of humility. Walking it out in your life is up to you. These are tender, vulnerable verses. So, quiet your heart and gently be real with God. He is transforming you into the likeness of His Son!

POSTURING DECLARATIONS

HUMILITY

I keep myself low before You. I live my life as a laid-down lover—a lover of God. Before You, Lord, I lay down everything I am. (Isa. 66:2)

I know what you are looking for: one who is humble and contrite in spirit and who trembles at your word and reveres your command. (Isa. 66:2)

Search my heart, Lord. Investigate my life and know my thoughts. Point out anything in me that offends You, and guide me along the path of everlasting life. (Ps. 139:23-24)

I take my day-to-day life—going to work, going to school, going to the grocery store—and place it before You as an offering. (Rom. 12:1)

As the highest form of worship, I place my body on your altar as a living sacrifice unto You. (Rom. 12:1)

So many in the world say, "I am rich. I don't need a thing." But I know differently. I am truly poor and blind and naked. I come to buy gold from You, gold that's been through the refiner's fire. I come to buy clothes from You, clothes designed in Heaven. And buy medicine for my eyes from You so I can really see. (Rev. 1:17-18)

Those whom You love You correct and discipline. That would be me. I ardently repent. (Rev. 3:19)

Whoever exalts himself will be humbled, and he who humbles himself will be exalted. (Matt. 23:12)

I clothe myself with humility toward other believers, because God opposes the proud but gives grace to the humble. I humble myself under God's mighty hand, that He may lift me up in due time. (1 Pet. 5:5-6)

I will not force my way or manipulate people to get a top position. I choose to put myself aside and help others get ahead. (Phil. 2:3)

God resists the proud but gives grace to the humble. Therefore, I humble myself under the mighty hand of God, that He may lift me up in due time. (1 Pet. 5:5-6)

In Christ Jesus, I posture as one gentle and humble in heart. (Matt. 11:29)

I humble myself like a child as I enter into Your Kingdom life. (Matt. 18:3, 4)

I rejoice because I am called a child of God. (1 Jn. 3:1)

I am concerned not only for my own interests but also for the interests of others. I take on the nature of a servant. I posture myself as a servant to all. (Phil. 2:3-7)

I am a foot washer. I continually posture myself in humility toward other believers washing my brother's feet so as to be like the Lord. (Jn. 13:14)

I am here to serve, just as the Son of Man came not to be served but to serve and to give His life as a ransom for many. (Matt. 20:28)

What does the Lord require of me? To act justly and love kindness and mercy and walk humbly with my God. (Mic. 6:8)

I choose to walk in obedience. I follow Your voice and walk in obedience. I love to serve You. (Phil. 2:8)

I fall prostrate before God. With each day, I remain lower still before Him, worshiping Him, loving Him, honoring Him, listening to Him, completely obedient to Him, and He pours out His wisdom and grace upon me. (Deut. 9:18)

I trust in You, Lord, with all my heart and lean not on my own understanding. In all my ways I acknowledge You, and You will make my paths straight. (Prov. 3:5, 6)

I serve the Lord with great humility and tears, having endured many trials. (Acts 20:19)

I meditate on Your Word day and night. In doing so, I am like a tree planted by streams of water which yields its fruit in season and whose leaf does not wither. Whatever I do prospers. (Ps. 1:2, 3)

I wait before You, Lord. I hope in You, and You energize me. (Isa. 40:31)

As a fragrant offering of fine perfume, I am broken and poured out before You, Lord. I give you the most valuable thing I have—my life, the essence of who I am. (Jn. 12:3)

Posturing Insights

- When you find you have difficulty believing a posturing verse, you most likely have believed a lie. Take notice: This is a place in your mind that needs to be rewired with God's truth. Write down the lie and then, after it, write the truth according to God's Word.

- You can pray, *"God, I'm sorry for believing the lie, and I break the agreement I have made with the lie. Forgive me. Heal the hurt place in my heart where the lie came in. Fill my heart and mind with Your truth as I speak Your Word. In Jesus' name, Amen."*

EXPERIENTIAL ACTIVATIONS

HUMILITY

Activation One

Now you are familiar with the foremost activation—daily posturing. Proclaim the humility verses for one week, first thing in the morning when you get up and right before you go to bed. Then, choose ten verses to speak at least once a day for thirty days. These truths will renew your mind and drop down into your spirit and become part of you.

Pride may come to discourage you, to keep you from binding yourself to humility. Right now, I see these verses like post-its all over your body. Do you sense what is happening? The word is life to you. God's word to Joshua (Jos. 1:8) was to "meditate on it day and night."

Read through all the verses aloud right now.

Activation Two

Play anointed worship music that really ministers to your heart and "lay low" before God. Put your body in a few different positions as you present your body as a living sacrifice before the Lord. Try being stretched out flat on the floor and kneeling and bowing before Him. Posture your heart as you posture your body. Use some of the posturing verses with which you feel strongly connected and say them to the lover of your soul. You can even meditate on what it means for you to be a living sacrifice. Really enjoy this. This is your time. Just you and your Creator.

Activation Three

In Acts 20:19, Paul said he was *"serving the Lord with all humility."* Google/look-up the meaning of humility. What does this word mean to you? Think of someone who exemplifies humility. How do you see humility demonstrated in this person's character? How is humility at work in your life?

Activation Four

Jesus came *"not to be served, but to serve and give His life as a ransom for many."* Every day we wash the feet of others when we serve and minister to them. Today, ask God for opportunities to demonstrate His heart of love and compassion toward people through simple acts of kindness. Want some ideas? Give out bottles of water. Smile. Tell somebody what a great job they are doing. I will often say, "Would you be offended if I prayed for you?" By asking permission, I have rarely been turned down. I tell them to close their eyes, and I pray a blessing over their lives. Or for whatever it is they need. It might be a need for healing in the body or heart, a better job, peace instead of anxiety, a closer walk with God. You get the idea.

PRAYER FOCUS

HUMILITY

Heavenly Father, In so many ways I've been led by my own desires—how I feel, what I want, what I think. I want to know: What is on Your heart, Lord? What is on your mind? What would You like us to do together? I humble myself before You, declaring that I offer myself as a living sacrifice. I am submitted to You and Your will. Lead me and teach me.
Amen

HEAVENLY WORD

Beloved, Choosing humility is to choose My Son's way. As you serve, I will enlarge your heart with My heart so that My love flowing through you will move you with compassion. Allow Me to interrupt your life when you see the needs of others. Be willing to stop. Be willing to love. Draw near to Me and let Me fill you with Who I Am.

"God is forever faithful and can be trusted..."

1 CORINTHIANS 1:9
PASSION TRANSLATION

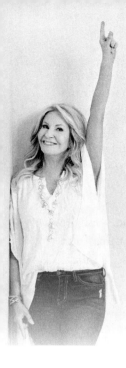

5

Completely Faithful
The Game Changer

Faithful: True to one's word, promises.
Steady in allegiance or affection; loyal; constant.
To be trusted, reliable.

You can't stop it. You cannot even hide from it. Run as fast as you want, but God's faithfulness is unrelenting. He meets you at every juncture. No matter how you mess up or how much pain your heart is in, His faithfulness is with you, nose to nose. He is true to His word, and His affections for you are 24/7. He feels your heartbeat and never abandons you. He is *completely* faithful. Completely means *lacking nothing!* He is committed to you all the time, in all ways and in all places. Recognize it. God's miraculous faithfulness is not of this world. No human comes even close.

Right now, say: *I believe You are completely faithful to me!* Miraculous hope is rising up.

About a week before my mother died, I had my final face-to-face conversation with her. I told her she was a good mother. She told me I was a good daughter. We were very close, and it pained me to think of life without my beloved mother. For a long time, we looked into each other's eyes. Finally, I said, *"I know I won't always have you ... but I've just got to trust God about this."* She agreed. We didn't know how much time we had left to spend together. We pledged to *trust* God—that He would be *faithful* to carry us through.

After she went to heaven, I felt God's strength. Did I grieve? Yes. And I cried. But I also felt amazing comfort. By the time we held her memorial service, I knew I had been given her mantle. Like Elijah and Elisha. I felt a cloak covering me like a weighty garment. At the memorial, two other people saw and confirmed my new mantle. What an incredible gift—far more valuable than any worldly inheritance. God not only helped me through the valley of pain, but He also bestowed on me far more than I had asked for or imagined— my mother's prophetic/evangelistic mantle. The Lord of my life once again proved to be extravagantly and miraculously faithful.

Our relationship with God is miraculous. *Every aspect of our identity is miraculous.* God's *faithfulness* is *miraculous.* His faithfulness reaches to the skies. Do you know anyone on earth who is as faithful as God? He knows everything going on in your life, and He *interacts* with you through His faithfulness. God is faithful to do what He says He will do. He is faithful to His Word. His very nature and character are unchanging. He fulfills all His wonderful promises. He promises He will take care of you. He is your Shepherd. He looks after your needs. He leads you into places of rest. He refreshes you and restores you. He guides you in paths of righteousness. He comforts you and protects you so you have *nothing* to fear. When all hell breaks loose, He sustains you. He anoints your head with oil. He pours so much into you that it overflows out of you! He makes sure that goodness and mercy follow you all the days of your life. He designed you to enjoy sweet, intimate fellowship with Him. He designed you to laugh—a lot. And when your enemy shows up, start looking around for the banqueting table. He prepares a table before you in the midst of your enemies! Nothing and no one in this world or in any other "religion" does this for you. Does this sound like Psalm 23? It is. He is your good and *faithful* Shepherd. Right here, right now.

Believing God is supernaturally faithful to guide you, help you, and love you is paramount to your faith. Believing in His faithfulness is a very big deal to Him. Huge. Of all the names God could have given, He first introduced Himself as "I AM." Doubting Him is like saying He is not almighty enough to see you through any hardship that comes your way. It is like saying He is not who He says He is. Choosing to believe that *He is,* while you are staring at the uncertainty of the future, compels you to acknowledge that God relentlessly invades your world with a heavenly reality where anything is possible. What else are you going to do? Where else are you going to go?

When most of us think of God's faithfulness, we think of His promises that have *already* been fulfilled in our lives. It is easy for us to acknowledge His faithfulness when we look back on our past and we see how God has brought us through the fire. The challenge occurs when we look at our current trials and the unknowns of the future. Our real faith is put to the test when we experience trials that can eat our lunch. The uphill journey of a trial—especially the most severe—is when we get to take an honest look at what's inside us—what we *really* believe.

God does not abandon you. He watches over you. He *watches* you. He sees your every move and is always working things together for your good. Guess what? In a trial, your faith is *tested*. Guess what again? God is supernatural. Guess what? God is an invader. Guess what? His faithfulness is supernatural. Guess what? He invades your circumstances with *supernatural faithfulness*.

Knowing He has already (past tense) given you hope ("I give you hope and a future," see Jeremiah 29:11) upon which to hang your faith during seemingly hopeless situations is a gamechanger. With your eyes fixed on God's unseen world of provision, your faith expands and your hope shines like a bright beacon in the darkness. Because you do not carry the outcome on your shoulders, people are drawn to the confidence and peace they see in you. When your situation does not turn out the way you want, you know He is faithful to work everything together for your good *anyway*! This is your purposeful posture of trust coupled with God's faithfulness producing *hope*. Boom! Gamechanger!

When we are *not* postured to believe that God is faithful, we can fall into the same trap the Israelites did: murmuring and complaining. They wandered around in the wilderness for forty years because they doubted He would be faithful to fulfill His Word. They did not step into what God already said was a done deal. Consider Hebrews. 3:8-11:

> *"During the time of testing in the desert,* [the children of Israel] ... *tested and tried me and for forty years saw what I did. That is why I was angry with that generation, and I said, 'Their hearts are always going astray and they have not known my ways.' So I declared an oath in my anger, 'They shall never enter my rest.'"*

The Israelites never entered the Promised Land. Israel witnessed how powerful God is and how He provided food and guidance for them, but they still doubted His goodness and complained any time something (in their eyes) went wrong. When the Promised Land was in sight, they were more impressed with their powerful enemies than God's power to give them the land. After all the ways the Lord had displayed His glory and good will toward them, they continued to disbelieve He would be faithful to give them the Promised Land!

What is *your* Promised Land? Are you postured as if it is a done deal—that you will, in fact, overcome the giants that are standing in your way? Many join the crowd of double-minded people who yell, "Hallelujah!" when everything is going great (in their eyes), only to cower in unbelief when things turn sour (again, in their eyes). Make up your mind about God *now*. Believe *now* in everything written in the Bible about God's character. It is not difficult—it is a *decision*. It's a simple shift of a mindset. Now is the time to take Him at His Word. Now is the time to choose to believe that He is reliable. Now is the time to purposefully posture in acceptance that He is faithful to YOU.

Don't wait until you are in the midst of a trial, finding yourself wondering if God is going to come through. Stop looking for Him to prove Himself to you. That attitude is coming from a place of doubt and unbelief in your heart. Determine in your heart to believe that God is faithful—now listen closely—even when the outcome of your trial isn't what you thought it should be. As you proclaim God's faithfulness, strongholds of unbelief will tumble down! You will find yourself in the heavenly realms with God's fidelity inscribed upon your heart.

God already has invaded, is now invading, and *will* continue to invade your life with His faithfulness. What is the fruit of His faithfulness in your heart? You learn you can *trust* Him. He is trustworthy because He is faithful to you over and over again.

Knowing, believing, and experiencing His faithfulness is the foundation for *trust*.

Each of us has a voice that matters. You are significant. Whether you speak up or not, what you believe will rise to the surface and be seen. Don't let your voice be a complaining and negative sound. Believing with ferocity in God's faithfulness will rock your life and cause you to stand up and release the roar of a mighty lion that shakes the earth!

Come on, lion! Stir yourself up and shake the earth by proclaiming who God is. Declare His very character to the earth—that He is faithful. Miraculously faithful! Each statement holds power when you speak of God's faithfulness with conviction. Warning: This is not for the faint of heart—this may actually *change* you.

POSTURING DECLARATIONS

COMPLETE FAITHFULNESS

God, You are completely faithful! You are reliable, and You are trustworthy! (1 Cor. 1:9)

You are true to Your word. Your affections for me are constant! (1 Cor. 1:9)

I can depend on You. And I do! (1 Cor. 1:9)

You cause everything to work together for my good. (Rom. 8:28)

Right now, You are working behind the scenes for me. I do not always see it, but I know You are. (Rom. 8:28)

You began a good work in me, and You are completely faithful to complete it. (Phil. 1:6)

You do all these amazing things for me that I cannot do! (Phil. 1:6)

God, You are faithful. Love and faithfulness go before You. (Ps. 89:14)

You offer a resting place for me in Your luxurious love. (Ps. 23)

You are faithful in keeping Your promises. (Heb. 10:36-37)

You are my good and faithful Shepherd. (Ps. 23)

You are faithful to take care of me. (Ps. 23)

You are my best friend and my Shepherd. I always have more than enough. (Ps. 23)

You promised to lead me into places of rest. And You do! (Ps. 23)

You promised to refresh me and restore me. And You do! (P. 23)

You promised to guide me in paths of righteousness. And You do! (Ps. 23)

The comfort of Your love takes away fear. (Ps. 23)

You promised to sustain me. And You do! (Ps. 23)

You anoint me with the fragrance of Your Holy Spirit! You pour so much into me that it overflows out of me! (Ps. 23)

Your goodness and love pursue me all the days of my life. (Ps. 23)

You designed me to enjoy sweet, intimate fellowship with You. (Ps. 23)

God, You are completely faithful, and You strengthen and protect me from the evil one. (2 Thess. 3:3)

God, You are faithful. You keep me steady and strong to the very end. (1 Cor. 1:8-9)

You are forever faithful and can be trusted. (1 Cor. 1:8-9)

You are faithful! You forgive me every time and cleanse me from all unrighteousness. (1 Jn. 1:9)

You are faithful to answer my prayers. (Ps. 143:1-2)

Great is Your faithfulness! (Lam. 3:23)

Your lovingkindness and Your compassions are new every morning! (Lam. 3:23)

Your love, O Lord, reaches to the heavens! Your faithfulness to the skies! (Ps. 36:5)

Your love stands firm forever. You established Your faithfulness in *heaven* itself! (Ps. 89:2)

O Lord, God Almighty, who is like You? You are mighty, O Lord, and Your faithfulness surrounds You! (Ps. 89:8)

You will never fail me. (Heb. 13:5)

You will never abandon me. (Heb. 13:5)

You have set me as a seal upon Your heart. You move on my behalf with passion like a raging flame. (Song 8:6)

All Your work, Lord, is done in faithfulness. (Ps. 33:4)

As a child of God, I know that You always hear me. (Jn. 11:42)

Your eternal Word stands firm in heaven. (Ps. 119:89-90)

Your faithfulness continues through all generations. (Ps. 119:89-90)

When I call upon You, You answer. (Ps. 91:15)

You are with me in times of trouble. (Ps. 91:15)

You deliver me and honor me. (Ps. 91:15)

You are completely faithful, even when I am not! (2 Tim. 2:13)

You are the author and finisher of my faith. (Heb. 12:2)

Because of Your love for me, You are faithful to discipline and correct me. (Heb. 12:6)

I am so thankful that You help me to stay on course! (Heb. 12:6)

I hold fast to Your promises, for You are faithful and always keep Your Word. (Heb. 10:23)

Great is Your faithfulness! (Lam. 3:23)

Great is Your faithfulness! (Lam. 3:23)

Great is Your faithfulness! (Lam. 3:23)

> ### POSTURING INSIGHTS
>
> - When you find you have difficulty believing a posturing verse, you most likely have believed a lie. Take notice: This is a place in your mind that needs to be rewired with God's truth. Write down the lie and then, after it, write the truth according to God's Word.
>
> - You can pray, *"God, I'm sorry for believing the lie, and I break the agreement I have made with the lie. Forgive me. Heal the hurt place in my heart where the lie came in. Fill my heart and mind with Your truth as I speak Your Word. In Jesus' name, Amen."*

EXPERIENTIAL ACTIVATIONS

TUNING INTO HIS FAITHFULNESS

Activation One

Giving into stress and forgetting that God is faithful is a battle all of us face. It is so easy to lose ground on this one. Many, many people do. We lose sight of God's faithfulness and look at our circumstances. We see the limitations of this natural world and step out of God's no-limitation world. God's faithfulness is left out of the equation.

How do we keep ourselves aware of God's perspective? A friend recently said to me, "Just keep looking down. Because that is the view from where you are seated—in heavenly places" (Eph. 2:6). When we posture, we speak from this "heavenly seated" place. We give voice to our agreement with heaven and speak from the heavenly realm perspective. People have told me they don't know if they should say some of the verses from the Bible because they do not see them as true in their life at the time. But this is exactly the purpose of renewing your mind—to bring your thinking into alignment with heaven. That means to dismantle old mindsets and replace them with new mindsets. Posturing is renewing your mind.

You know what to do: Posture in the Completely Faithful Declarations of this chapter twice a day—once in the morning and once at night. Do it right when you get up and right before you go to bed. After one week, choose ten verses to continue to speak for thirty days. Now you are really transforming mindsets! Declare to the atmosphere around you and in you of God's faithfulness. Be like the persistent widow and don't give up (Lu. 18:1-8). In doing so, you prepare yourself for heavenly dreams as well as beginning your day with a heavenly perspective.

Activation Two

God promises that He will never leave or forsake you (Heb. 13:5). He has always been right by your side through thick and thin. Think of a time when you felt as if God deserted you but later realized He was with you all the time. Often, we see a bigger picture weeks, months, or even years later. Think of a challenging situation you face right now. Yes, God is at work in the middle of your current trial, just as He was in the past. Why is God's faithfulness a gamechanger?

Take a moment to get quiet and tell yourself that God is helping you right now. In doing so, you are purposefully choosing to take a scriptural mindset. With this activation, say to the Lord throughout the week, *"I know You are helping me with this trial—because You are faithful!"*

Activation Three

Renewing your mind is to come into agreement with God's unrelenting faithfulness and allowing His faithfulness to become more deeply rooted in your being. Yet God is also calling *you* to be faithful. I often tell those I mentor that God is more concerned with *how* you do what you do than *what* you do. In speaking to the church in Smyrna in Revelation 2:10 (Passion Translation) the Lord says:

> *"... remain faithful to the day you die and I will give you the victor's crown of life."*

Integrity matters. Being honorable and keeping your word matters. Holding fast to your faith matters. Your faithfulness matters. Consider the following affirmation:

"I belong to God. He chose me and set me apart to Him. Before the heavens and the earth, I proclaim over my life: God is completely faithful to me! And I choose faithfulness. I, myself, choose to be faithful in all I do."

Ponder it in your heart. Right now, proclaim the words. As you speak them, anoint yourself with oil. (Hand lotion will work too. Once I used toothpaste when there was nothing else!) This can be a significant point of remembrance in your life.

Activation Four

Craft a personalized psalm heralding the Lord's faithfulness. What has He done for you in the past? What is He doing for you now? What do you believe He will do for you in your future? How does this reflect His nature and character?

Activation Five

Throughout this study, we have immersed ourselves in God's faithfulness to us. What about our faithfulness to God? And our faithfulness to people? Faithfulness is a fruit of the Spirit (Gal. 5:22-23). Daily, we take a stance for faithfulness and choose how this fruit will mature in us. We choose to be faithful to God. We choose to be faithful to others and grow in our faithfulness. Faithfulness is not a have-to—it's a want-to. Even a get-to.

> *"The one who manages the little he has been given with faithfulness and integrity will be promoted and trusted with greater responsibilities. But those who cheat with the little whey have been given will not be considered trustworthy to receive more. If you have not handled the riches of this world with integrity, why should you be trusted with the eternal treasures of the spiritual world: And if you have not been proven faithful with what belongs to another, why should you be given wealth of your own?"* (Lu. 16:10-12)

Think about your faithfulness. Consider ways you have managed with faithfulness and integrity what you have been given. What are they? How are you faithful to God? How about others? Write a list of ways you are and can be faithful.

PRAYER FOCUS

AMAZING FAITHFULNESS

Heavenly Father, You are so faithful! When I
think about how You have always been there for

me, it shatters my fears about the future. As I go through difficult trials, You are faithful to work all things together for my good. You call me to be faithful as well. I say, Yes! I also am faithful. I will continue to be faithful for all my days, and You shall give me the crown of life. I keep my promises—I am a person of integrity. I rely on You, and You strengthen me. You are faithful to watch over me! With every breath I take, You are faithful.

Amen

HEAVENLY WORD

Dear One, Remember what John saw? He saw heaven open, and there before him was a white horse whose rider is called Faithful and True. That's My identity: Faithful and True. That's Who I Am. I created you and planned you. Surely, I can take care of you. I do not ever sleep—I am always watching over you! I Am FAITHFUL and TRUE!

REVELATION 19:11;
PSALM 139:13; PSALM 121:4

"Trust in the Lord completely, and do not rely on your own opinions. With all your heart rely on him to guide you, and he will lead you in every decision you make. Become intimate with him in whatever you do, and he will lead you wherever you go."

PROVERBS 3:5-6
PASSION TRANSLATION

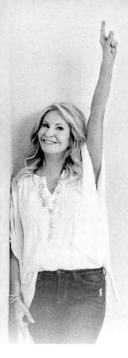

6

Trusting God
Rely on Him

Trust: confidence, assurance, and reliance in God
and all that He is and all that He says.

He looked up from the pathology report, "It's positive." My husband took my hand. "And I know what you have ahead of you." Sure, he knew. He was a medical doctor and had been treating cancer patients for the previous ten years. Most of them were women with a breast cancer diagnosis—like me.

I never thought it would happen to me. After all, I had been the office chaplain. I was the one who prayed for cancer patients. I saw miracles. I saw people healed. How could this happen to me?

I experienced a visceral reaction I never would have suspected: I felt shame. That's right. I was ashamed and embarrassed that I, a Christian minister, one who believed in healing and who ministered in signs and wonders could have a breast cancer diagnosis. I believed I was immune to such things. I went to God with my mixed bag of emotions and self-deprecating thoughts, and I handed them over. I needed to set my feet on the rock.

If you want to draw closer to God, you are going to have to trust Him … with *everything*. Trusting God means you are confident in Him—that He is *good*, that He *loves* you, and that He is working everything together for your good. The challenging part of trust is that He doesn't conform to our timetable. We have deadlines; He sees a bigger picture. We see obstacles; He sees breakthroughs. We see ways we think things could or should work out; He persuades us to forego leaning on our own understanding.

When we go through really tough trials—and it feels like all we can do is hold tight to the hem of His garment and fly through the storm—He is watching. *Will she still love Me and trust Me even if the answers don't come the way she wanted?* Trust is a decision that no matter what situation you find yourself in, you are determined to believe that God is trustworthy and that He is good.

As your faith grows stronger, your trust becomes more pervasive. Now you trust Him with your finances, your family, and your future. Every detail of your life is entrusted to Him. Sometimes He reveals tucked-away places where you are white-knuckling it and still trying to hold on and handle things yourself. With great tenderness, you loosen your grip, and your trust expands. Where are you headed? Trusting without limits.

To fully trust means that in the depth of your being, you are unwilling to give up, give out, or give in. Trust compels you to step into a miraculous world. Why? Because you trust God for miraculous intervention. Trust believes in things not seen. Trust believes that the supernatural hand of God is at work behind the scenes. Trust knows He is working all things together for your good because you love Him (Rom. 8:28). Trust watches.

The most meaningful season of our faith is not when answers to prayer are manifesting right and left, but when we continue believing even though we are not yet seeing any fruit. Many times—during severe trials, when I cannot see the end in sight—I pound my fist and say, *"Lord, whatever happens, I'm not giving up! God, I trust You! You are the One directing my path!"* Faith is complete trust that, in the middle of that trial, God is *for* you.

We have postured in God's faithfulness. Now it is time to position ourselves in limitless trust. Being faithful is what *He* does; trust is what *we* do. Perhaps you feel as if you have little faith or trust. Not to worry. Everyone is given a measure of faith that will grow. Just like the tiny mustard seed turns into a huge tree, your trust-life increases in size (Matt. 13:31-32; 17:20).

God is alive; your faith is coming alive. Bible verses on trust provide powerful encouragement for you to better comprehend faith and the trust walk. You will not be the same next week as you are today— the tree absolutely will grow! You are unfolding, budding, and blossoming. Don't concern yourself with how small the seed is right now. Go by what is true. Speak with confidence, knowing you are extravagantly loved and highly favored.

When you purposefully take steps to transform your thinking, it won't be just a head thing. It will revolutionize your heart. So, get ready for a revolution as you proclaim these verses with all your heart! Here we go ... soaring in the realm of trust without limits!

POSTURING DECLARATIONS

TRUST WITHOUT LIMITS

I trust You, Lord, with all my heart. I do not rely on my own understanding. In all my ways I acknowledge You, and You direct my path. (Prov. 3:5-6)

You are far greater than my circumstances, and You work all things together for my good. (Rom. 8:28)

I trust You, Lord, with my future. (Jer. 29:11)

Even when things don't turn out the way I want, I still trust You. (Prov. 3:5-6)

I trust that You care about every detail of my life. (Matt. 6:26)

I trust that Your grace is sufficient. God, Your ability is at work in me, and Your power is made perfect in my weakness. (2 Cor. 12:9)

Lord, I trust that You are with me wherever I go, always watching over me. (Ps. 23)

Though I walk through the valley of the shadow of death, I will fear no evil for You are with me. (Ps. 23)

My mind is focused on trusting You, therefore You keep me in perfect peace. (Isa. 26:3)

Blessed is the man who believes in, trusts in, and relies on the Lord. That's me! (Jer. 17:3)

My hope and confidence is in the Lord. (Jer. 17:3)

Because I trust in You, unfailing love surrounds me. Every time I turn around I find that You love me. (Ps. 32:10)

Without faith it is impossible to please God. I have faith. I trust in God. (Heb. 11:6)

I am confident that You reward those who earnestly and diligently seek You. I am a diligent seeker! You are rewarding me right now! (Heb. 11:6)

I live my life by faith. I am sure of what I hope for and certain of what I do not see. (Heb. 11:1)

I know I have faith because God has dealt to everyone a measure of faith. (Rom. 12:3)

Faith comes by hearing, and hearing by the word of God. I speak the word of God; I increase my faith. My faith is growing every day. (Rom. 10:17; 2 Thes.1:3)

I am fighting the good fight of faith, trusting God all the way. (1 Tim. 6:12; 2 Tim. 4:7)

The message of faith is on my lips and in my heart. From the depths of my heart, I proclaim: *I trust in the promises of God!* (Rom. 10:8)

I boldly believe for whatever I ask for in prayer, that I have received it, and it will be mine. (Mk. 11:24)

Speaking by faith in the name of Jesus produces mighty miracles. (Jn. 14:14)

Trials come to prove that my faith is genuine. As fire purifies gold, my faith will be tested. My faith is far more precious than gold. I am up to the test. I will not waver. I trust God. (1 Pet. 1:7)

When my faith is tested, it stirs up power within me to endure all things. (Jas. 1:3)

During a trial, I get to see exactly where my faith is. When my faith is tested, endurance and patience have a chance to grow. (Jas. 1:3)

The righteous shall live by faith. I have complete confidence in God and His ability to supply all things. (Rom. 1:17)

I believe God for signs, wonders, and miracles. I act on my faith, for faith without works is dead. (Jas. 2:26)

I am fully persuaded that God is able to do immeasurably more than all I ask or imagine. (Eph. 3:20)

I am confident that His supernatural power is alive and working in me! (Eph. 3:20)

I put on the complete armor of God, and when warfare hits, I take up the shield of faith with which I extinguish all—not some or a few—but *all* the devil's fiery darts. (Eph. 6:13, 16)

POSTURING INSIGHTS

- When you find you have difficulty believing a posturing verse, you most likely have believed a lie. Take notice: This is a place in your mind that needs to be rewired with God's truth. Write down the lie and then, after it, write the truth according to God's Word.

- You can pray, *"God, I'm sorry for believing the lie, and I break the agreement I have made with the lie. Forgive me. Heal the hurt place in my heart where the lie came in. Fill my heart and mind with Your truth as I speak Your Word. In Jesus' name, Amen."*

EXPERIENTIAL ACTIVATIONS

ACKNOWLEDGING GOD IN ALL YOUR WAYS

Activation One

When circumstances in our lives challenge our faith and trust in God, we must already be prepared to fight the good fight of faith. A warrior doesn't prepare when he/she goes into battle—he prepares long *before* the battle. We prepare when we tenaciously align our thoughts with heaven. Our thoughts then become power thoughts. Declare these personalized verses out loud twice a day for a week. Release them over the circumstances of your life.

You are becoming an intentional speaker, saturating yourself with truth. Declaring that which is true transforms you inside. The fruit of your inner work will manifest in your daily life. Becoming aligned with how God sees you transforms your life. You will experience your faith and trust in God increase markedly!

Choose ten verses and continue to declare them for the next thirty days. A new lifestyle is forming. Keep the momentum.

Activation Two

The Israelites told stories of God's mighty miracles to their children and to their children's children. Events were commemorated by naming locations, people, and cities after miracles and encounters with God. They made sure all God had done for them would be remembered for generations to come.

Ask the Holy Spirit to show you major trials you have faced and how you chose to trust God. Close your eyes and relive what God did for you. Commemorate God's intervention on your behalf by taking the time to write about the event and what He did for you. Keeping a record of all God has done for you strengthens your faith. You chose only one event, but I'm sure if you meditated on it, you would see how vast His involvement in your life has been. (There will be a place in the workbook for this.)

Activation Three

Go with a friend on a "trust walk" in your neighborhood. This activation may challenge you, which is why I suggest you do this with someone with whom you feel a level of trust. Hold your friend's hand, close your eyes, and let him/her lead you on a walk. With your eyes closed, touch flowers, trees, buildings. You can even try walking fast. Consider how it feels to no longer be in control. This exercise would be a starting place in the natural realm. But the God of all creation has wonderous places and revelations to show you.

> *"No eye has seen, no ear has heard, no mind has conceived what God has prepared for those who love him"—but God has revealed it to us by his Spirit. The Spirit searches all things even the deep things of God"* (1 Cor. 2:9-10).

The Holy Spirit is the Revealer, and He reveals to us the deep things of God. We are on a miraculous adventure! As we let go of our preconceived ways of experiencing the world and open our spiritual senses to the Lord, heavenly adventures ensue. Your life with God is a supernatural "trust walk." You have been posturing about having a more intimate relationship with God. He is the One who takes you on spiritual walks and shows you His treasures in heavenly realms. All of this is a biproduct of developing an intimate relationship with the Father.

Activation Four

Read Philippians 1:6 in a few translations. God began a good work in you and will continue developing that good work until the day of Christ Jesus. What specific areas in your character are you trusting God to bring to full completion in you? What specific ways are you doing what you need to do to cooperate with God's work in you?

What dreams and visions are you trusting Him to fulfill? Quickly, jot them down. Again, how are you doing your part? Many Christians think all they need do is sit back, wait, and do nothing. But this is a relationship. He calls us to work together with Him. Remember: Faith without works is dead. Using olive oil (or whatever you have on hand), anoint yourself as a symbolic way of consecrating yourself as one who trusts God daily. You can do this as you pray the Trust Prayer written below.

PRAYER FOCUS

MIRACULOUS TRUST

Jesus, You are faithful and true. Forgive me for doubting You and taking matters into my own hands. I place my hands on my head and proclaim before You that I am posturing myself as one who trusts You. Your timetable is beyond my comprehension. When your ways don't make sense to me, I still trust You. I won't rely on my own limited understanding. I boldly let go and live a life of simple trust.
Amen

HEAVENLY WORD

Dear One, Be confident of this: I began a good work in you, and I will carry it on to completion. I am able to do far more than you can ask or imagine. So think big and trust Me. I am watching over every detail of your life. I sent you the Holy Spirit to help you. He is called the Helper—that's Helper with a big "H!" Rely on, call on, lean on My Spirit as your Helper. You are never alone. I am always with you. In this moment, I am with you. I know where you are, and I am with you.

PHILIPPIANS 1:6; EPHESIANS 3:20;
JOHN 14:16-20

"You will guard him and keep his in perfect and constant peace whose mind [both its inclination and its character] is stayed on You, because he commits himself to You, leans on You and hopes confidently in You."

ISAIAH 26:3 AMP.

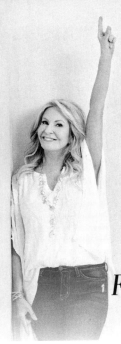

7

Miraculous Peace
Fear and Anxiety Cannot Have You

Peace: a state of rest, quietness
and calmness; perfect wellbeing; an absence of strife.

"*I will get through this. I am going to make it. I have hope, and I have a future. I'm going to make it.*" My voice sounded small. Even squeaky. It was the middle of the night, and for the first time, I was completely alone. All my friends and family had left. "*This is way too soon for me to be all alone,*" I thought. But everybody had a life to return to, jobs, families, and planned vacations. My husband was gone—living in heaven. And it was only me—and God. I knew it. I had nowhere to go, no one to call, nothing I could do. With my head half buried under the covers, I knew I had to take hold of my one and only lifeline. I had to. I must align my thoughts with heaven. I had to see myself through God's eyes. Riding on a wave of His word was my only hope. My mind had to be steadfast, trusting in Him, believing Him, relying on Him.

Over the ensuing weeks, my voice grew stronger. *"I have hope and I have a future."* In the middle of the night, when loneliness was pressing down on me, I said this over and over. During the day, those words kept me moving forward. The Holy Spirit was strengthening me as I agreed with heaven about my future. I am not saying it was easy. As you can imagine, it wasn't. Hey, I had been married over thirty years. I had to fight for God's promise of peace. But I chose to hold on to the hem of His garment while I struggled through the storm. Peace about my having a future without my husband dropped from my mind down into my spirit. Excitement came. Joy came. Enthusiasm came. I started working on my next book.

You may be asking something like this: *If Jesus came to give me peace, why does it seem so hard to receive sometimes?* Two reasons. First, real peace comes only from God. It is a promise in His promised land of promises. What does that mean? That means it is attainable, but we must fight for it. We must overcome the giants of opposition. We must persevere. Remember this: God said the promises are yours— you can well take the land. Posture yourself to fight *from* victory, not *toward* victory.

Second, we have an antagonist, a thief that comes to steal, kill, and destroy our peace. His main tactic: fear. The battle over fear is right between your ears. Then the emotions come in. If you let the fear go unchecked, sickness can emerge. Let me give you an example of how quickly it happens.

Peter boldly entered God's supernatural world and walked on water. He fixed his eyes on Jesus and defied his circumstances. The moment his focus switched from Jesus to the circumstances, fear-inducing thoughts invaded his mind. *What am I doing?! These waves are huge! I'm going to drown!* In a split second, Peter was back in the world of limitation, with fear gaining the upper hand. He began to sink. He had no peace. Right on the heels of fear came worry.

Plain and simple: The robber of peace is fear. Fear immobilizes us. It keeps us from moving forward with our jobs, relationships, finances—and, most importantly, it keeps us from entering God's supernatural world where ANYTHING is possible. Even walking on water. Fear paralyzes us and gets us to make "safe" if not inferior decisions. It robs us of the joy and breakthrough that comes from being courageous and taking risks. It keeps our dreams at bay. Fear can come from a harassing spirit that does not come from God. When our *thoughts* come into agreement with it, this spirit gains a stronghold in our lives that will hold us in bondage.

Worry and anxiety are symptoms of fear. Anxiety torments a person about scary things that could happen. It robs people of sleep and the ability to focus during the day. Anxiety about what we don't have, could have, or could lose can consume our minds. It brings peace-stealing thoughts like these: *Your future looks bleak. You're going to fail. You're not going to survive this. You'll never get this bill paid off.* And those thoughts can assault every one of us.

So, what are you going to do when the attack hits? As soon as we realize it's just an attack on our peace, it's time to lasso our thought life. When anxious thoughts aren't dealt with, anxiety becomes a way of life. It becomes a stronghold in your mind. I'll bet you can think of people you know who are constantly worried about something. Anxiety is a trap, an illusion right from the pit of hell. Anxiety reveals where our focus is—either on Jesus or on the storm.

You want to know what else steals your peace? Feeling rushed, behind the eight ball with deadlines, and basically not having enough time to get everything done you believe you need to do. Often, I wish I had more time to get everything done. It seems like the prime hours of the day go by so quickly. Can you relate? When our "to do" lists don't get done, we feel stressed. When our circumstances go south, we often complain. When people do wrong by us, we become hurt and angry. When doors of opportunity don't open, we get discouraged.

All of this leads us to one place: FEAR! And that fear puts a doormat out for anxiety. Will it ever end? It's doubtful. We will continue to be busy and have trials the rest of our lives. Even so, God makes one thing clear: Jesus came to give us peace! He has plans for each of us—and He will fulfill those plans. Time does not concern Him. He stands outside time. He has made the way for you to overcome every obstacle and find a supernatural peace as you do it. Here is the BIG KEY:

God gives you enough time to do everything He has called you to do.

Living our lives like we don't have enough time to our day can make us feel inadequate and incompetent. We just run around like a chicken without a head! I strongly believe this is a tactic of the enemy: to convince us to put so much on our plate that we get overwhelmed and feel bad about ourselves. Time is valuable. A precious commodity. Why do you think the devil wants us to run out of time? So we do not give any of our time to God! That's right. The jig is up. I cannot tell you how many have told me they are too tired to get up early to pray. Too tired to spend time with God. Your time is a battlefield. Recognize it.

Most feelings of fear and worry generate from a place where we are not acknowledging the reality that God is with us. Peace is a person, and His name is Jesus. In Psalm 23, the psalmist poetically states that God is with us when we walk through the valley of the shadow of death. Wow, that's intense! Death is all around, casting its shadows, but God is with us. There really is nothing about which to be afraid. Even death has lost its sting!

Psalm 23 goes on to describe peace to the max. Here the Lord makes us to lie down in lush green pastures and rest beside still waters. Sounds peaceful, right? He even prepares a dinner for us in the presence of our enemies. Now that *has to be* supernatural peace. Who can relax enough to eat dinner while his enemies are glaring and jeering at him? When all hell breaks loose, right in the eye of the storm, God can keep us in a place of perfect peace. And as He does, He is serving us filet mignon and a chocolate torte. Ha! Now that is some table service. So, when life becomes difficult, posture your attitude and start looking around for the banqueting table.

To begin the process toward possessing supernatural peace, enter God's heavenly realms and develop a new mindset. A river flows from God's throne with healing for the nations. When your eyes are on Him and His provision, this river will flow into and through you to bring His peace to your life and your circle of influence. As your thought patterns get realigned, the demonic strongholds that oppose you are weakened, and God's Kingdom is established. Well, come on! What are you waiting for? Jump into the river. Let's shatter some strongholds and proclaim sweet peace!

POSTURING DECLARATIONS

PEACE IS YOURS

Lord, I choose to keep my mind focused on You, and You will keep me in perfect peace. (Isa. 26:3)

Peace like a river is flowing through me. (Isa. 48:18)

I speak peace over myself. I proclaim peace over my life. I bind myself to peace. (Gal. 1:3)

To my brothers and sisters I proclaim, "Grace and peace to you! Grace and peace to you! Grace and peace to you from God our Father and the Lord Jesus Christ!" (Gal. 1:3)

You guide my feet one step at a time down the path of peace. (Lk. 1:79)

You have provided peace for me, Lord. Not a false peace that comes from the world, but a real peace that comes from heaven. My heart will not be troubled, nor will I be afraid. (Jn. 14:27)

I cast all my worries, all my anxieties, all my concerns upon You, because You care for me. (1 Pet. 5:7)

When I do not know what to do, my eyes are on You, Lord! (2 Chron. 20:12)

I am postured to not worry about things in my everyday life. My Heavenly Father is looking out for me. If His eye is on the sparrow, how much more is He watching over me. (Matt. 6:25)

I seek God's Kingdom above all else, and everything else will be added to me. (Matt. 6:33)

The God of peace shatters everything that is the antithesis to peace. He will crush Satan under my feet! (Rom. 16:20)

Because I trust You, I am unshakable. I am deeply at peace. In this world I experience difficulties and challenges. But I take heart, because You have overcome the world! (Jn. 16:33)

I will not worry—I will pray. With thanksgiving, I present all my requests before You. Your supernatural peace is not of this world. It transcends all my human understanding and

places a guard around my heart and my mind.
(Phil. 4:6,7)

The mind controlled by the Holy Spirit is life and peace. Holy Spirit, take control! (Rom. 8:6)

Jesus, You paid a great price so I could have peace. You were pierced for my transgressions, You were crushed for my iniquities; the punishment needed for me to have peace was upon You, and by Your wounds I am healed. I receive Your peace! I receive Your peace! I receive Your peace! (Isa. 53:5)

I let the peace of Christ rule in my heart. (Col. 3:15)

I pray, and You answer me. You deliver me from all my fears. (Ps. 34:4)

The Kingdom of God is alive in me with righteousness, peace, and joy in the Holy Spirit. (Rom. 14:17)

The fruit of the Spirit is love, joy, peace, patience, kindness, goodness, faithfulness, gentleness, and self-control. Fruit of the Spirit, grow large in me. Peace, grow in me! (Gal. 5:22, 23)

Jesus, You are the Prince of Peace. Your name is called Wonderful, Counselor, Mighty God, Everlasting Father, and the Prince of Peace. (Isa. 9:6)

I take Your yoke upon me and learn from You for You are gentle and humble in heart, and I will find rest for my soul. (Matt. 22:29)

The Lord restores my soul. (Ps. 23:3)

I will lie down and sleep in perfect peace, for You alone, O Lord, make me dwell in safety. (Ps. 4:8)

When I lie down, I will not be afraid; when I lie down, my sleep shall be sweet. (Pr. 3:24)

Lord, You have made it clear that You will not, will not, will not leave me or forsake me. (Heb. 13:5)

As I wait on You, Lord, I find new strength. I soar on wings like eagles. I run and do not grow weary. I walk and do not faint. (Isa. 40:28, 29, 31)

I dwell in the shelter of the Most High. I abide in the shadow of the Almighty. You deliver me from dangerous traps and deadly diseases. You shield me with Your faithfulness. I am covered by Your wings. You are my refuge and my fortress, My God, in whom I trust! (Ps. 91:1-4)

Because I have made the Lord my refuge, the Most High my dwelling place, no evil will befall me. No plague will come near my house. (Ps. 91:9-10)

I will not fear the terrors of night or the dangers of day. I will not be intimidated or fear what everyone else fears. Ten thousand people may fall at my side, but I will remain untouched! (Ps. 91:5-10)

God has given His angels charge over me to guard me in all my ways. They will bear me up in their hands, and I will not strike my foot against a stone. I will tread upon and trample the lion and cobra! (Ps. 91:11-13)

Because I have set my love upon You, You will deliver me. (Ps. 91:14)

Because I have sought to know Your name, You will set me securely on high. (Ps. 91:14)

I will call upon You, and You will answer me; You will be with me in trouble; You will rescue me and honor me. With a long life You will satisfy me, and show me Your salvation! (Ps. 91:14-16)

I have hope, and I have a future. (Jer. 29:11)

I will go out in joy and be led forth in peace! I am led by Your peace! Lead on! Lead on! Peace, lead on! (Isa. 55:12)

POSTURING INSIGHTS

- When you find you have difficulty believing a posturing verse, you most likely have believed a lie. Take notice: This is a place in your mind that needs to be rewired with God's truth. Write down the lie and then, after it, write the truth according to God's Word.

- You can pray, *"God, I'm sorry for believing the lie, and I break the agreement I have made with the lie. Forgive me. Heal the hurt place in my heart where the lie came in. Fill my heart and mind with Your truth as I speak Your Word. In Jesus' name, Amen."*

EXPERIENTIAL ACTIVATIONS

PEACE

Activation One

Proclaim the Peace is Yours verses twice a day for seven days. You are establishing a daily routine. Begin your day saying the personalized verses and again at night before bed. After one week, choose ten verses to include in your thirty-day posturing list.

Activation Two

What is stealing your peace? Make a list of things in your life that cause you fear, stress, or anxiety. What are your top three places of concern? Write your list.

Read over your list and ask yourself, *"Do I want to keep these worries and fears?"* As you can see from my story at the beginning of the chapter, you do not have to remain subject to your inner turmoil. Your starting place is to simply give your list to God. Cast it all on Him. The Passion Translation of 1 Peter 5:7 reads as follows:

> *"Pour out all your worries and stress upon him and leave them there, for he always tenderly cares for you."*

In other words, give it all over to Him. Why? Because He cares for you. The Lord tells us not to be anxious. He is literally saying that we are to transfer the burden of our soul over to Him. This is huge. Do not take it lightly! Seriously, *transfer all your burdens to Him!*

He then tells us to be thankful and pray. At that point, He will help us. God Himself will put a *guard* around our minds and hearts so we can have peace. This is the answer you have been looking for. Guarding your heart and mind is not a small matter! *"...the idea is not merely that of protection, but of inward garrisoning as by the Holy Spirit"* (Vines, p. 284). A garrison of peace is also a big deal! It is a body of troops stationed in a fortified place. Talk about protection. God is saying if you give your anxiety over to Him, then He will put troops around your mind. And your heart! His guard is an inward protection. Philippians 4:6-7 describes the whole enchilada:

> *"Do not be anxious about anything, but in everything, by prayer and petition, with thanksgiving, present your requests to God. And the peace of God, which transcends all understanding, will guard your hearts and your minds in Christ Jesus."*

There are more places in the Bible instructing us not to worry. Take your anxiety list into the secret place and give it to God. Burn it, wad it up, throw it in the trash—whatever it takes. Give Him your list. Thank Him for the inner guard around your heart and mind that keeps peace within you. Take a couple deep breaths and read back over the posturing verses.

Activation Three

Most of us have certain people who always tend to bring chaos and drama into our lives. Evaluate how much access God wants you to give them into your life. Is God really calling you to them? If so, what boundaries do you need to enforce? Keep in mind, true peace does not involve making treaties at the expense of giving away pieces of your life. If you have the workbook, you will have a place to write your perceptions.

Activation Four

A trigger point for worry often springs from trying to juggle an overloaded schedule. Remember, you have enough time to do everything God has called you to do. If you are overloaded and worn out, look at what's on your plate. Take your big plate to the Throne Room and ask God what stays and what goes. We must pace ourselves as we run the race. Yes, we can all have extra-busy seasons—but that can't be the norm or you will burn out. It's when we are overly tired that fear and anxiety taunt us. Setting some schedule boundaries is a good first step to recapturing peace.

PRAYER FOCUS

PEACE

Dear Lord, I need Your peace to reign in my life. Ever-increasing peace. I truly believe You are bigger than all my troubles. I am choosing not to worry or be stressed out. I trust you and release all my anxieties to You. True peace is mine. I have peace like a river running through me!
Amen

HEAVENLY WORD

Beloved, One of My names is the God of Peace. Jehovah Shalom. I am the Source of all peace. My peace I give to you. It is not the kind of peace the world offers—My peace is real ... and deep ... and life-changing. Come close to Me and let Me deliver you from the enemies of your soul. I will guard your heart and your mind by giving you a peace that transcends all understanding. I will wrap a blanket of peace around you, for I am the God of all comfort. Do not let your hearts be troubled and do not be afraid. I am always with you. In the middle of all storms, I am there with you.

JUDGES 6:24; JOHN 14:27;
PHILIPPIANS 4:6-9;
2 CORINTHIANS 1:3-4;
PSALM 23

*"But let him who boasts boast about this:
that he understands and knows Me..."*

JEREMIAH 9:24 NIV

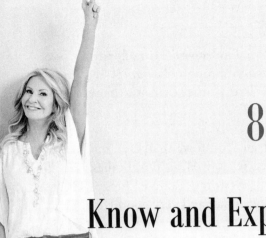

8

Know and Experience God
Personal, Intimate and Real

Know: to progressively become more deeply
and intimately acquainted with God

Sunlight filtered through the cottonwood trees dangling over the Big Wood River. A small group, including my husband, waited on the grassy shore. One after another waded into the clear, cool, mountain water to be baptized by the pastor. I sat on a blanket and watched. I'd been sprinkled when I was four. I didn't think I needed to do it again. As glorious a day as it was, my heart was heavy. I understood so little about God. Turning to the woman next to me, I said, "I don't know how to know God." She looked at me and said nothing. She was in the same boat as I: longing to know about God, but not knowing how to get there—to Him.

Many of us have bumbled along, trying to get closer to God. We've listened to sermons and read the Bible, but deep inside, we know that we don't know Him. Not the way we know a good friend. Or even a not-so-close friend. We don't always trust Him with complete confidence. And that's because we don't know who He is. In a very personal way, we don't know His character. And we are not sure how to get closer. Not really. How does God reveal Himself to us? Two primary ways: through His *actions* and through His *names*. His names reflect His character—what He is like. Rather than list the names of God, let's look at His character.

We know that He's the God of all Comfort, that He's our Peace, and our Healer, healing our hearts as well as our bodies. He is also our Provider, our Shepherd, Restorer, Refuge, Judge, Hope, Righteousness, and our beloved, personal, and very good Papa. He is a consuming fire, destroying everything opposed to His holiness. He is holy—completely. He is personally involved with you to the degree that you will let Him. Everything about you holds His attention. As you get to know Him, He *engages* with you. To engage means to attract and hold fast, to occupy the attention of, to become involved with and secure for aid.

He gives you grace to accomplish all He calls you to do. His grace and mercy endure forever. He is jealous for you and loves to spend time with you. He loves to guide you and reveal new things to you. He leads you into places of rest and places of war. He enables you to succeed at both. His banner over you is love. With Him, you can overcome any enemy. He is God Almighty—nothing is impossible for Him.

He is love, and He pours out His love on you day and night, with kisses from heaven. He is the One who sees you and knows everything about you. He is the Most High—nothing, no one, is higher. He has all power, all authority, and all sovereignty. He is the Ruler of all things. He is the Alpha and Omega, the beginning and the end. He shows up in your life all day long—and throughout the night. He is the stay-up-late-and-talk-about-everything friend. *Look* for Him and *engage* with Him.

Let me give you a simple example of engaging with God: This morning, I sat quietly with Him. I talked with Him about the chapter I am working on, and I asked Him for the ability—the grace—to write the revelation He's given me in such a way that it would bring inspiration to the one reading it. He gave me guidance on how to proceed, and off I went, trusting in His grace to write.

The heart of this chapter is not only to *know* God, but most importantly to *experience* God. To experience is to personally encounter, undergo, meet with, or feel.

> *"Eternal life means to know and experience you the only true God, and to know and experience Jesus Christ, as the Son whom you have sent"* (Jn. 17:3 Passion Translation).

You can know of God and about God, but it is in your spiritual DNA to *experience* God. To know Him is to have intimate, experiential knowledge of the highest level. You are unique, and God encounters you in ways that are personal to you. He gets you and desires for you to experience Him. You can look at an airplane, but it is another thing to ride in that airplane. You don't have someone else's experience in that airplane—you have your own personal experience in the airplane. You can watch a convertible coming down the street, but to experience riding in one with the wind, the blue sky, the sunshine ... ahhhh!

You can know about a milkshake, but the cold, delicious taste is a stand-alone experience. You can gaze upon the beauty of a rose, but to experience the fragrance is incomparable. God is way beyond all the natural world offers. Your miraculous identity experiences a miraculous God!

You can know that God loves you, but the deep, lasting, inner transformation comes when you *experience* God's love. His love is not a platitude or memorizing a verse. God is relational. He pursues you; you pursue Him. He is alive in your life. Right now, say, *"You are so active in my life! I am recognizing Your presence in my life more and more every day!"*

Experiencing God is intimately receiving from Him. Even now, as you read this, the thickness of His presence surrounds you. Even now, your spiritual eyes are opening. Stop reading for a minute, take a breath, and sense His presence. If you have been speaking the declarations in this book, you are becoming deeply postured in your miraculous identity and purposefully entering into greater intimacy with God.

How has He engaged with you in the past twenty-four hours? I asked this of one of the young women I mentor. She told me that the day prior she was in a very stressful situation. Right in the middle of it, she felt The God of All Comfort with her. She also told me that morning she'd had a garage sale and sold everything she had hoped to sell. That was God the Provider. The God of favor. The God of grace. He shows up revealing many facets of who He is. God is continually engaging with us. He continually reveals Himself through all the attributes of His character. We just have to slow down and recognize Him.

You probably won't like to hear this, but a primary block that keeps us from recognizing Him is complaining. Just like the Israelites and ten of the twelve spies, complaining keeps us from obtaining and living in what He has already said is ours. All of them saw the same thing, but ten of the spies viewed the Promised Land from a worldly viewpoint—not God's viewpoint. What they saw were insurmountable obstacles. Complaining is viewing our circumstances from a worldly perspective. To see God engaging with us requires us to see from heaven's perspective.

Pursuing the knowledge of God and experiencing Him is like a magnetic force (for lack of a better term) that *glues* us to His perspective. Knowing by experience what He is like enables us to *trust* and *see* from heavenly places. We are going to shift our posture completely to that of a pursuer. It is vital that we grow militant in our proclamations. The verses you will speak in first person are not only powerful declarations, but also a form of worship. Take these before God as worshipful proclamations. Knowing and experiencing God is at the heart of knowing your identity.

POSTURING DECLARATIONS

KNOWING AND EXPERIENCING GOD

Jesus, I continually long to know and experience You more fully. (Phil. 3:10)

My determined purpose is that I may know You. (Phil. 3:10)

I consider everything a loss compared to the surpassing greatness of being intimately acquainted with You. (Phil. 3:8)

I desire a deeper relationship with You. (Phil. 3:8)

More and more, I am perceiving You and recognizing You. (Phil. 3:8)

More and more, I understand You more fully and clearly. (Phil. 3:8)

I am growing in knowledge of You because I experience You. (Phil. 3:8)

I am encountering You every day. (Phil. 3:8)

I think of You through the watches of the night. (Ps. 63:6)

There is no one like You. (Isa. 46:9)

Wherever I go, You are there! (Ps. 139:7-10)

Like Job, I say, "I had heard of You by the hearing of the ear, but now my spiritual eyes *see* You." (Job 42:5)

Early will I seek You. My whole being thirsts for You. (Ps. 63:1)

To know You is to encounter You. (2 Cor. 3:16-18)

I receive revelation from You. Through the Scriptures, You implant Your thoughts into my mind. (1 Cor. 2:9-12)

The only thing I can boast in is this: that I understand and know You. (Jer. 9:24)

I recognize how You are engaging with me. (Jer. 9:24)

I directly discern Your character. (Jer. 9:24)

You are the Lord who practices kindness, justice, and righteousness in the earth. (Jer. 9:24)

I wait on You. I am developing sensitivity to Your presence and promptings. (Ps. 25:4-5)

Show me Your ways; teach me Your paths. Lead me in Your truth and teach me! (Ps. 25:4-5)

I wait on You. What an honor to wait on YOU!! I set aside time to be alone with You. (Ps. 25:5)

Like Moses, I say, "Lord, show me Your glory." I've received Your promises, seen Your power, experienced Your presence. I'm looking for YOU! YOU—more intimate knowledge of YOU! (Ex. 33:18)

Your compassion toward me is so strong it never fails. How could I not want You back? (Lam. 3:22-23)

And You desire me! You are jealous for me! A holy jealousy! And a passionate commitment to me. (Deut. 4:24)

You enable me to do and complete the work to which You have called me. (Zech. 4:9)

This is eternal life: to know You, the only true God, and Jesus Christ, whom You sent. (Jn. 17:3)

This is to perceive, recognize, become acquainted with, and understand YOU! (Jn. 17:3)

POSTURING INSIGHTS

- *Breaking Agreements with Lies:* When you find you have difficulty believing a posturing verse, you most likely have believed a lie. Take notice: This is a place in your mind that needs to be rewired with God's truth. Write down the lie and then, after it, write the truth according to God's Word.

- You can pray, *"God, I'm sorry for believing the lie, and I break the agreement I have made with the lie. Forgive me. Heal the hurt place in my heart where the lie came in. Fill my heart and mind with your truth as I speak your Word. In Jesus' name, Amen."*

EXPERIENTIAL ACTIVATIONS

KNOWING AND EXPERIENCING GOD

Activation One

Daniel 11:32 is a very enlightening passage. It says, *"...the people who know their God shall be strong, and carry out great exploits."* To fully enter the arena of supernatural, mighty exploits, we need to have our identity solidly built on our knowledge of who God is. We need to know what He is about. We must know His character and nature. Begin taking aggressive action through posturing in Knowing and Experiencing God.

Proclaim the verses in the above section twice a day. The best times are first thing and last thing: when you rise in the morning and before bed. Allow them to saturate your being. After one week of proclaiming the verses, choose ten to proclaim for the next thirty days.

Activation Two

We are becoming more in tune to how God is engaging with us. Engage means to occupy the attention or efforts of a person. Ask the Holy Spirit to show you how God has engaged with you in the past twenty-four hours. What do you see?

Activation Three

Think about God's nature and character. Consider His names. Read over God's characteristics listed earlier in this chapter. During major upheavals and huge triumphs in your life, how have you experienced these characteristics of God?

Activation Four

To have a profound activation requires a set-apart time for a heart-to-heart communion with God. Psalm 42:2 reads, *"My soul thirsts for God, for the living God. When can I go and meet with God?"* Take the posturing verses and the attributes of God to your secret place and pour yourself out—heart, soul, and mind.

PRAYER FOCUS

PURSUING GOD

O Lord, I want to know and experience You.
Really know You, like King David and Apostle
Paul did. I want to know the power of Your
resurrection. I choose to be more sensitive to how
You engage with me in every day. I participate
with You. I enjoy You. You know everything
about me—I long to know everything about
YOU! I love You! Come away with me. Come
quickly!
Amen

*"O God of my life, I'm lovesick for you in this weary wilderness.
I thirst with the deepest longings to love you more, with cravings
in my heart that can't be described. Such yearning grips my
soul for you, my God!"* (Ps. 63:1 Passion Translation)

HEAVENLY WORD

Dear One, I love being pursued by you. I loved
that when Paul and Silas were in jail, they pursued
Me. I loved how David got up early and pursued
Me. I love to see you going after a deeper, closer,
more intimate fellowship with Me. Look at Me,
and fall into My eyes. I am in you and you are in
Me. With your eyes fixed on Mine, I draw even
closer to you. The love between us is like a blazing
fire many waters cannot quench. Place Me like

a seal over your heart. Know that nothing can separate you from My love!

ACTS 16:25; PSALM 63:1; JAMES 4:8;
SONG OF SONGS 8:6-7; ROMANS 8:39

"Call to Me and I will answer you and show you great and mighty things, fenced in and hidden, which you do not know (do not distinguish and recognize, have knowledge of and understand)."

JEREMIAH 33:3 AMP.

9

Getting Pictures from God
God Invades Your World

Picture: a visual representation of a person, object, or scene. A mental image, however produced.

The room around me disappeared. A vivid picture of mythological Atlas carrying the world on his shoulders filled my mind. I stared at the enormous burden carried by this one man. The image came alive as I saw the world lift from his shoulders. I watched in amazement as I simultaneously felt a very heavy weight lift from *my* body. I did not know of the burdensome weight I bore until it was gone. Tremendous love and joy flooded me. What was happening to me? I felt fantastic! Like a whole new person! This was the day I invited Jesus into my heart. I was eleven.

My understanding of the Atlas picture God had given me grew as I matured in my relationship with Jesus. Atlas represented *me*—carrying the weight of the world. The world represents the sphere of sin a person carries, having not received the saving grace of Jesus available to all. The lifting of the world from Atlas's shoulders speaks of God's redemption and the magnitude of God's love. Jesus came to redeem His creation and set us free from the bondage of a fallen world. The moment I asked Jesus to forgive me for my sins and thanked Jesus for dying on the cross and to come into my heart, His love and joy ravished me. For years, that picture from God continued to minister to me.

One of the ways God speaks to us is by giving us pictures. Sometimes we also receive immediate revelation. Sometimes revelation comes over time. Sometimes the image is only a quick glimpse, while at other times the picture can be a more lasting image. For example, my husband lost the registration to a car he wanted to sell. He looked everywhere and could not find it. Finally, he prayed and asked God to show him where it was. He received a glimpse of his pink slip and where it was located. Confidently, he went to the location, found the slip, and sold the car.

God shows us "great and mighty things fenced in and hidden" of which we have no knowledge. Whether He speaks in a whisper or with a quick glimpse of a picture, He is teaching us to become sensitive to His leading. I could give you many examples of times I did not follow a glimpse from heaven. And I could tell you of many times I did. I could also tell you of many times I asked God about something and received no picture at all. The point is to grow in intimate friendship with Him so you become more and more familiar with His voice and His ways. In Jeremiah 33:3, God tells us to ask Him, and He will show us great and unsearchable things. He will show us things we would not otherwise know or see.

When you become a Christian, you are to purposefully renew your mind, right? What does your mind contain? Thoughts and images. Renewing your mind includes renewing images as well. Some mistakenly believe that the imagination is bad and images are not to be trusted. This is just one more area the devil has endeavored to steal from the body of Christ. As taught in *The Real You*, your mind is a great battlefield. Satan wants to control it. The war is not only for your thoughts, but also for the *images* in your mind. The place in you where images are planted belongs to God. The Bible teaches us to pull down vain imaginations. Why? So wrong thoughts and *images* are demolished, and that same place—your mind—is to be filled with God thoughts and God images.

When I pray for someone, I posture in a place of expectation. I expect God to answer, and many times He gives me a picture. Often a word of knowledge will accompany the picture. For example, last week I prayed with a man who is fighting cancer. I felt strongly that God was drawing this man to Himself, and I saw a magnet, which the Holy Spirit called a love magnet. I had received both a word of knowledge and a picture. Let me add that sometimes I will get a picture and not know what it means. In this case, I did not know what the picture meant. Often the person I am praying for knows exactly what it means. The man understood the love magnet picture, and it greatly ministered to him.

Every Christian can receive pictures from God, and I would be bold enough to say *does* receive pictures from God. The purpose of pictures is to receive greater insight into matters that are on God's heart. Pictures encourage you, give you hope, and guide you in the right direction. With more insight, we can become aware of and cooperate with God's purposes. The Holy Spirit is the ultimate Revealer, and He reveals things to us through thoughts and pictures. The *gifts* of the Holy Spirit often manifest in us also by way of thoughts and images. Revelation through images permeates the gifts of the Spirit.

When you receive a picture or have a vision, the heavenly realm opens up to you. Here is a great example of heavenly realms opening and revealing God's intentions and purposes. In 2 Kings 6:15-17, the heavenly realm opened up to Elisha's servant. The servant was afraid when he saw an enemy army with horses and chariots surrounding him and Elisha. Elisha told his servant not to be afraid and prayed that God would open his servant's eyes to see into the heavenly realms. The Lord opened the servant's eyes, and he saw the hills full of God's army.

In the second chapter of Acts, Peter quotes the prophet Joel, delivering a prophetic word describing the great outpouring of the Holy Spirit. Peter said God is pouring out His Spirit with dreams and visions and prophetic insights on His people.

> *This is what I will do in the last days—I will pour out my Spirit on everybody and cause your sons and daughters to prophesy, and your young men will see visions, and your old men will experience dreams from God. The Holy Spirit will come upon all my servants, men and women alike, and they will prophesy. (Acts 2:17-18)*

Throughout the Bible, we see God bestow pictures and dreams on His people. In Acts 10:11-12, Peter had a vision that made the way for the gospel to be given to the Gentiles. In Acts 9:10, the Lord called to Ananias in a vision. The entire book of Revelation is filled with pictures and visions.

Before we start posturing, we are going to pray for your mind to be consecrated to the Lord. To consecrate means that you declare your mind is sacred, set apart and dedicated to serve Him. Next, simply believe God is interacting with you. Ask what it means. Even go to the Word to search it out. Study biblical references about what He has shown you. In addition, you will recognize the peace of the Holy Spirit. He leads you with His peace. At this point, I want to make clear that I am not talking about conjuring up images or trying to force God to move by picturing something over and over in your mind. God initiates the pictures He gives you.

Pray: *Lord God, I consecrate my mind to You. My mind is sacred and set apart for You. I dedicate my mind to serve You. I pray the Jeremiah 33:3 prayer, asking you to show me great and mighty things I would not otherwise know. I want to see through Your eyes! You are the Revealer. I now activate my spiritual sense of seeing. Teach me how to connect with*

You through my spiritual senses. I purposefully posture in my miraculous identity. In Jesus' Name, Amen

After you have asked for a sanctified, clear, and seeing mind, trust the very next (first!) thing God shows you. It might not make sense to you. It may even seem obscure, and you might think it came from you. Remember, He shows you things you would not otherwise know! So, often it won't make sense. Consider Peter's vision of the clean and unclean animals. It did not make sense at first. Take what He shows you and, like Peter, ask God about it.

The way we posture will be slightly different for this chapter. Just like Elisha, we will ask the Lord to open our eyes and show us pictures of what He wants us to see. We will posture ourselves in verses where God showed things to biblical characters, and then how God reveals His plans and purposes to us. Remember, God even opened a donkey's eyes to see into the spirit realm (Num. 22:21-34). The posturing truths God speaks to His people with pictures and visions and dreams will encourage you and stir up your spirit to be ready for God to drop pictures into your spirit. Co-laboring with God is an integral part of the awesome, fun adventure we are on with God!

POSTURING DECLARATIONS

GETTING PICTURES FROM GOD

God *reveals* what eye has not seen and ear has not heard and what has not entered into the heart of man. (1 Cor. 2:9-10)

God unveils and reveals such things to me. (1 Cor. 2:9-10)

Holy Spirit, You reveal to me profound revelations of God. (1 Cor. 2:10)

You show me things hidden and beyond man's scrutiny. (1 Cor. 2:10)

I have received the Holy Spirit that I might realize and comprehend and appreciate the gifts bestowed on me by God. (1 Cor. 2:11)

I welcome the revelations of God's Spirit into my heart. Because I am a spiritual being, I examine, investigate, inquire into, and discern all things. (1 Cor. 2:14-15)

I have the mind of Christ, and I hold the thoughts—the feelings and purposes of His heart. Lord, teach me more about having the mind of Christ! (1 Cor. 2:16)

The eyes of my understanding are being enlightened. I call forth the eyes of my understanding to be opened! (Eph. 1:18)

The Holy Spirit lives in me and is with me, and He teaches me all things. He takes what is of God and reveals it to me. (Jn. 14:26)

I cast down vain imaginations that are not from heaven. Lord, place heavenly inspired images in my mind. Mind, be filled with God's purposes! (2 Cor. 10:4-5)

I ask You to show me unsearchable things I would not otherwise know. You have given pictures to your servants throughout the Bible. And You give them to me. Lord, let me remind You of the mighty things You have shown us! (Jer. 33:3)

You showed a pillar of cloud by day and a pillar of fire by night! (Ex. 13:21)

To the Israelites, the glory of the Lord looked like a consuming fire! (Ex. 24:17)

Because of a dream, Gideon knew he could prevail over his enemy! (Judges 7:15)

On Pentecost, You showed us tongues of fire! (Acts 2:3)

You showed Stephen God's glory, and Jesus standing at God's right hand! (Acts 7:55)

You showed Peter a sheet lowered from heaven, containing unclean animals! (Acts 10:11-12)

You opened the eyes of Your servants on the road to Emmaus. (Lk. 24:31)

You pour out Your Spirit on all people. Your sons and daughters prophesy, your young men see visions, your old men dream dreams. (Acts 2:17)

I earnestly desire and cultivate spiritual endowments—the gifts of the Spirit—especially that I may prophesy, interpret the divine will and purpose in inspired preaching and teaching. (1 Cor. 14:1)

You will show wonders in the heavens above and signs on the earth below. (Acts 2:18)

In the morning, I present my requests before You and wait expectantly. I expect you will show me things. I anticipate Your faithfulness. (Ps. 5:3)

POSTURING INSIGHTS

- When you find you have difficulty believing a posturing verse, you most likely have believed a lie. Take notice: This is a place in your mind that needs to be rewired with God's truth. Write down the lie and then after it, write the truth according to God's Word.

- You can pray, *"God, I'm sorry for believing the lie, and I break the agreement I have made with the lie. Forgive me. Heal the hurt place in my heart where the lie came in. Fill my heart and mind with your truth as I speak your Word. In Jesus' name, Amen."*

EXPERIENTIAL ACTIVATIONS

PICTURES FROM GOD

Activation One

Proclaim the Pictures from God verses twice per day for seven days. Begin and end your day saying the personalized verses. Then, choose ten to include in your thirty-day posturing list. If, for some reason, you have not been speaking the verses, start now. Do not be hard on yourself. Take a breath and begin with these verses.

Activation Two

Read 2 Kings 6:8-14. God supernaturally allowed Elisha to know what the king of Aram was speaking in the privacy of his bedroom. Elisha *heard* what was being spoken. Maybe he even *saw* what went on in the king's quarters. We do not know how many of Elisha's spiritual senses were discerning the spirit realm in this event.

Read verses 15–17. Elisha could see into the spirit realm. God revealed that the hills were full of horses and chariots of fire. We know Elisha was not afraid, because he told his servant not to be afraid. When your spiritual eyes are opened and you see from God's perspective, you will experience changes inside. Fear goes. Anxiety goes. Limiting mindsets go.

Elisha prayed for his servant's eyes to be opened to the realm of the Spirit, and his eyes were opened. Now it's your turn. Ask the Lord to open your eyes. Just ask. Like you asked God to save you and fill you with the Holy Spirit. The how, when, what, why, and where is up to God. It may be now and it may be later. What you are doing is saying "YES!" to God for your eyes to be opened.

Pray: *Father just as Elisha prayed for his servant's eyes to be opened, I ask You to open my eyes that I might see in the realm of the Spirit. I want to see what You are doing and see things from Your perspective so I can come to a place of higher revelation. You said for me to fix my eyes on what is unseen. I do so now. I yield my eyes to You now. Open my spiritual eyes to the realm of the unseen. According to Your purposes and Your plans for me, I ask for all you have for me—including more visions, more dreams, more revelations, and more supernatural encounters with You. In the Name of the Lord Jesus Christ, I pray. Amen.*

Activation Three

Practice "seeing with God." During your prayer times, ask Him to give you insight about something that has been on your heart. As you sit quietly in His presence, wait and watch. When He impresses you with a picture, write it down.

Ask the Lord to reveal what the picture means. He may tell you right away, or He may want you to press in to Him for more understanding. Sometimes I just "know" what the picture means. Other times, my understanding of the picture unfolds over time. Go to the Bible and look up all references that talk about the picture. Watch for confirmations. A confirmation can be found in anything: a billboard, a song, a sunset, a movie (Yes! He has spoken to me in movies so much that I took notes in the dark!) or in what seems to be an idle conversation. Watch.

Activation Four

Your spiritual sight is only one of your spiritual senses. Activate all your spiritual senses to not only see, but also to hear, feel, smell, and taste. Hebrews 5:14, Passion Translation, says, *"But solid food is for the mature, whose spiritual senses perceive heavenly matters."*

I teach a lot from Romans 12:2, but this verse is preceded by Romans 12:1—a crucial verse about presenting our entire selves as a living sacrifice to God. Amplified says, *"...to make a decisive dedication of your bodies [presenting all you members and faculties] as a living sacrifice, holy (devoted, consecrated) and well pleasing to God, which is your reasonable (rational, intelligent) service and spiritual worship."* I take it to mean *all* your senses.

Pray: *Father, I activate all my spiritual senses. I want to be fully engaged with you! Activate all my spiritual senses to not only see, but also to hear, feel, smell, and taste. I offer my whole self as a living sacrifice, holy and pleasing to You—which is my spiritual worship. Amen.*

Activation Five

Read 1 Corinthians 2:10-16 and John 16:13-15 in a few translations. The Holy Spirit guides us, speaks to us, and reveals things to us. To reveal means to make known something that was previously secret or unknown. It is to bring a hidden thing to the open. The Holy Spirit makes things known that are unknown or hidden, and in doing so He helps us navigate through challenging waters. He is a revealer of divine secrets. Think of a specific situation you need God to guide you through. Using these verses, talk to Him about your situation. Ask Him to reveal hidden things about this situation.

PRAYER FOCUS

SEEING FROM HEAVENLY REALMS

Dear Lord, There is a place in me where You speak to me through images. I consecrate my imagination for Your Kingdom. Open my spiritual vision so I can discern what I cannot see with my physical eyes. I ask You for revelation, and I also ask for wisdom. You opened the eyes of Elisha's servant to see into the spiritual realm around him. I posture myself to see what You want me to see. I posture myself to be more in sync with Your supernatural dimension. Open the eyes of my heart!
Amen

HEAVENLY WORD

Beloved, I call you friend, and it is to my friends that I reveal my secrets. You have heard my people are destroyed for lack of knowledge. You have heard that without vision, my people perish. To be in on My plans and purposes, you must have revelation. A sanctified imagination responds to My Spirit. Spend time with Me. Ask of Me. I pour out My Spirit on all people. You will prophesy; you will see visions; you will dream dreams. I will show you great and unsearchable things you would not otherwise know.

JOHN 15:15; HOSEA 4:6; PROVERBS 29:18;
ACTS 2:17; JERIMIAH 33:3

"David was greatly distressed; for the men spoke of stoning him, because the soul of them all was bitterly grieved, each man for his sons and daughters; but David encouraged and strengthened himself in the Lord his God."

1 SAMUEL 30:6 AMP.

10

Encourage Yourself in the Lord

To Encourage Yourself is to Strengthen Yourself

Encourage: be strong, courageous, strengthened,
established, firm, mighty.

Quite a few years ago, my husband and I filed for bankruptcy. Our large medical practice had a barely functioning heating-and-air-conditioning unit ignored by a neglectful landlord. Patients who normally sat for a couple hours having an IV, didn't want to come in under such adverse conditions. We were forced to close. As we prepared to file, discouragement beckoned us. Here I was—a ministry leader, speaking at churches and conferences—facing bankruptcy. How could this happen when I had been devoting myself to serving the Lord? I felt embarrassed, defeated, and flat out discouraged. I looked for consolation and encouragement from other leaders. Surprisingly, a few responded critically, looking at me as if my choices or behaviors had caused the problem. So, I refrained from confiding in most of my peers. Many days I had no one to call, no one to tell me that everything was going to be all right. It was just me … and God. On one of these occasions, the light bulb went on. Wasn't King David in a similar situation?

David and his men had just returned home to Ziglag only to find their city had been burned down and all their wives and children kidnapped. After they cried out all their tears, David's men began talking about assassinating him. David was metaphorically circling the toilet, stripped of everything—his reputation, his self-will, his close companions with whom he'd fought side by side. He could have given up and succumbed to the notion that all was lost, including his life—but he didn't. Instead, he *encouraged* himself in the Lord. What? How did he do that? He was in a gigantic, no-way-out-of-this mess!

With his back against the wall and death in his face, a pep talk of persuasive words of worldly wisdom wouldn't cut it. David chose the God way out. David encouraged himself *in the Lord*. And in doing so, he made himself *strong* in the Lord.

The root of the word encourage is "to fasten upon." How did David fasten himself upon the Lord? What did he do? I firmly believe he told himself all about God's greatness and goodness. He wasn't just speaking words of worldly encouragement. He was stepping into God's world and standing in the path of God's very breath, where true encouragement can transform a person. He remembered all the miracles he'd seen God do, all the promises God had spoken to him, and all the intimate hours he'd spent with the Lord God. He might have picked up some of his own poems and proclaimed them aloud. He "fastened" himself to the Lord until he was strong and courageous again.

> *"Have I not commanded you? Be strong and of good courage; do not be afraid, not be dismayed, for the Lord your God is with you wherever you go."* (Joshua 1:9 NKJV)

When Joshua was about to enter the Promised Land, the Lord told him not only to continually meditate on His word, but He also told Joshua to speak the Word. Exactly what we are doing in this course! Then the Lord told him not to be afraid but to be strong and courageous.

In Joshua 1:9, "be strong" is the same Hebrew word used in 1 Samuel 30:6, when David encouraged himself. When he encouraged himself, he literally made himself strong in the Lord. When you encourage yourself, you strengthen yourself. This is why it is vital that you proactively *encourage* yourself. You cannot let this slide. You haves to decide now to make this inner change. Your hidden journey will dramatically shift and even accelerate with ongoing encouragement. To overcome devastating trials and tribulations, your survival depends on your posture of self-encouragement.

Each of us can go through very difficult seasons. Maybe you're in one now right now. We have two choices: Give up or get strong. When there is nowhere to turn and hardship seems to be overtaking you, how do you encourage yourself? I asked a group of women this question, and without hesitation one of them said, "I don't!" I have a sense this statement is true for most of us: We rarely think about encouraging *ourselves*. Today, all this is going to change. You are going to stand in the path of God's breath and feel His words of encouragement surging through you.

According to the New Testament, prophecy is speaking forth God's mind and counsel. When we prophesy, it is not always futuristic, but often a declaration of that which is not known by natural means. We are speaking not from an earthly viewpoint—but from God's viewpoint. When we prophetically speak to someone, we are strengthening, encouraging, and comforting him with God's truth (1 Cor. 14:3). Likewise, we can do the same for ourselves. I feel I am "prophesying" to myself when I speak God's word over myself. I am strengthened and encouraged!

The way you will use the "Encourage Yourself in the Lord" section will be a bit different. For this posture, you will speak directly to yourself. Not about yourself. To yourself. Stand in front of the mirror, look into your eyes, point to yourself, and in a strong voice proclaim the personalized posturing verses. That's right. It's just you, the Holy Spirit, and the mirror. Tune in to how Holy Spirit activates these truths deep in your being as you speak them forth. If your voice starts out weak as a kitten, don't cave. You've got to start somewhere. You will probably not believe everything you speak. Be sure to address the lies and break your agreement with them. After a few days in front of the mirror, pace around your house and speak over yourself. Then keep going back to the mirror. This takes discipline and perseverance. But many times, for many of us, it is the difference between life and death. Just like David, you have an enemy who wants to take you out. Encouraging yourself is the way to truly live strong. Let's go!

POSTURING DECLARATIONS

ENCOURAGE YOURSELF IN THE LORD

You are going to make it! (Rev. 12:11)

You will fulfill everything God has called you to do! (Phil. 1:6)

I prophesy to you—you are strong and courageous! (Josh. 1:9)

You have resurrection life in you! (Eph. 3:20)

The power of the Holy Spirit lives in you! (Acts 1:8)

I command your spiritual eyes to open to greater revelation! (Eph. 1:18)

I call forth the gifts of God in you! (Matt. 25:14-30)

I speak to your spirit and say, "Rise up! Stand strong!" (Eph. 6:10)

I command the sleeping giant in you to arise!! (Eph. 5:14)

Warrior bride, arise! (Isa. 60:1)

I speak to all the places in you God is now calling, "Wake up!" (Eph. 5:14)

God can do ANYTHING!! And He can do ANYTHING through YOU! (Phil. 4:13)

Don't go by what you see! Don't go by circumstance! Don't go by feelings! (2 Cor. 5:7)

All of heaven is backing you up! (Matt. 28:18)

Almighty God is going ahead of you and making the way for you! (Ps. 5:8)

Step into a world of vision and color and sound! Step into the sounds of heaven! (Rev. 4)

Step into the supernatural realm! You are a supernatural being! (2 Cor. 5:17)

Right now, I break off demonic assignments against you! (Matt. 28:18)

I break off crazy thoughts, in Jesus' Name! (Matt. 28:18)

I break off self- hatred, in Jesus' Name! (Matt. 28:18)

I break the assignment of the destroyer, in Jesus' Name! (Matt. 28:18)

You have a sound mind! God has not given you a spirit of fear, but of power, of love, and of a sound mind! (1 Tim. 1:7)

You will get over your past! (2 Cor. 5:17b)

You have a future! There is hope in you! You have hope and a future! (Jer. 29:11)

You have authority given to you by Jesus! (Lk. 10:19)

I prophesy—multitudes will come into the Kingdom of God through your life! (Acts 1:8)

Every place you put your feet, YOU OWN! (Josh. 1:8)

You are an atmosphere changer! (2 Cor. 2:15)

Through Christ in you, you dominate the spirit realm around you! (Col. 3:27)

So get over yourself! You are an overcomer! (1 Jn. 4:4)

You will not quit! You will not give up! (Rom. 12:21)

Look at your situation and say, "I AM AN OVERCOMER!!" (1 Jn. 4:4)

You have the victory already! Before it manifests, you have the victory! (1 Jn. 4:4)

Stand up! Satan is a liar and a thief and an accuser. But greater! But greater! But greater is He who lives in you! (1 Jn. 4:4)

Listen to me: God can turn anything around! (Matt. 19:26)

I speak complete health over you! (1 Pet. 2:24)

Immune system, I command you to be strong! (1 Pet. 2:24)

I prophesy—you are an overcomer! (1 Jn. 4:4)

Strength from heaven flows through you! (2 Cor. 12:9)

You shall prevail! And win! (1 Jn. 5:4)

I command hope to rise up in you. Confidence— rise up! Boldness—rise up!! (Heb. 4:16)

I speak into your entire being: you are so loved by God. (Jn. 3:16)

Outrageously loved with an everlasting love! (Jer. 31:3)

Live strong!! Stand firm! (Josh. 1:9)

You are going to make it! (Rom. 8:31-32)

POSTURING INSIGHTS

- When you find you have difficulty believing a posturing verse, you most likely have believed a lie. Take notice: This is a place in your mind that needs to be rewired with God's truth. Write down the lie and then, after it, write the truth according to God's Word.

- You can pray, *"God, I'm sorry for believing the lie, and I break the agreement I have made with the lie. Forgive me. Heal the hurt place in my heart where the lie came in. Fill my heart and mind with Your truth as I speak Your Word. In Jesus' name, Amen."*

EXPERIENTIAL ACTIVATIONS

ENCOURAGING YOURSELF

Activation One

To transform the way we talk to ourselves, we must replace words of self-limitation and discouragement with biblical words of encouragement. This means we purposefully take *action*. That's the beauty of this activation. You now have a solid tool in your hand to strengthen yourself and find ongoing encouragement. Speak the posturing verses to yourself twice a day. Begin in front of the mirror. Pointing to yourself at times for emphasis. Then, after a few days, pace and speak over yourself. For one week. Do this first thing when you get up and last thing before bed.

Choose ten verses to continue speaking for the next thirty days. By the end of this course, you will have 100 verses. It sounds like a lot, but it will take you about twenty minutes. Don't stress. The Lord told Joshua to think about and speak the word day and night. You can do this. The more you do, the stronger you become. Often, I take the verses on my morning walk and then I will keep them in the car so they are easily accessible to me throughout the day.

After thirty days, you can change out the verses. Yes, posturing (renewing your mind) is a lifelong affair. Remember, renewing your mind *transforms* you. But *you* are the one who does the act of renewing. It is for *you* to do.

Activation Two

Ask Holy Spirit a very important question: *"Holy Spirit, what words do I need to say to myself? What do I need to hear?"* When I have taught identity intensives, I have directed people to ask Holy Spirit this question. Over and over again, I see each person know what he/she needs to hear. It will be something positive and encouraging that perhaps you have a hard time saying to yourself. It could be something like, *"You're beautiful. You're lovable. You're smart. Life is worth living. You have heavenly gifts within you to share with the world."* Look deep into your eyes in the mirror and say this Holy-Spirit-inspired truth.

Activation Three

Stop for a minute and think of a challenging situation you are currently dealing with in your life. Ask Holy Spirit what you could say to yourself that would be encouraging. Ask Him what verse reflects this. Write the verse and say it to yourself right now. What is going on deep inside? Is there another verse? Go for it! Is He healing your heart? Enjoy it! Get out your Bible and look up verses that deal with what you are going through.

Activation Four

When you encourage yourself by aligning yourself with every Word that proceeds from the mouth of God, you make yourself strong. Read Luke 4:1-14. How did Jesus face temptation? Do you think we could view this as how Jesus encouraged Himself and made Himself strong?

PRAYER FOCUS

ENCOURAGING MYSELF

Dear Lord, You have told me I am planned, accepted, and wanted. You have created me to overcome. You have forgiven me. You love me. I am highly valued. I am a new creation with a new identity. A miraculous identity! Today, I choose to encourage myself with Your Word. You speak to my heart and tell me such wonderful things. I don't want to negate Your Word by saying negative, discouraging things to myself. I am sorry for every negative thing I've spoken over myself! There is no discouragement in heaven. No critical spirit in heaven. As I take a stand to encourage myself, I am strengthened. I dig in my heels and purposefully declare words of heavenly encouragement!
Amen.

HEAVENLY WORD

Beloved, I give you hope and a future! Yes! You have a future! Do not live in worry and fear. Your future is in My hands. Trust Me—even when the outcome is not what you think it should be. Trust that I know things you do not. As you seek Me, the Holy Spirit reveals deep things to you that are on My heart. I have planted hope in you. Seek Me with all your heart. I will be found by you. I take great delight in you. I rejoice over you with singing. I dance over you. I am always encouraging you and restoring you and embracing you. Engage with Me and take Me at My Word. Just agree with Me about yourself. Speak My Word! My Word is like a hammer that breaks a rock in pieces. My Word is a lamp to your feet and a light to your path!

JEREMIAH 29:11-14; ZEPHANIAH 3:17;
LUKE 4:4; JEREMIAH 23:29; PSALM 119:105

ABOUT LINDA

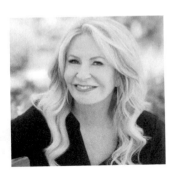

Linda Breitman Ministries, located in San Diego, California, is a nationally recognized force behind women's groups, faith-based ministries, and church-based Bible Studies. She has been a featured speaker for AGlow Conferences, International Women's ministries, Jubilee Conferences and a featured guest on Christian Broadcast News, Igniting a Nation, Money Talk with Melanie, The Hard Question with Blanquita Cullum and many more radio and TV programs.

She is the author of The Real You Identity Courses and has spearheaded the Prophetic Intercession Training Schools and Dangerous Women Activation Seminars.

She hosts a weekly podcast which features authors, leaders, and speakers in the church community; leaders defeating child abuse, sexual assault, ending teen homelessness; providing job opportunities for military spouses, and tackling the many social issues that canvas our society. To hear Linda's latest podcast please visit: www.lindabreitman.com

For More Information about Linda Breitman, visit:
www.lindabreitman.com

Let's Connect....

Facebook: www.facebook.com/LindaBreitman

Twitter: www.twitter.com/LindaBreitman

Instagram: www.instagram.com/LindaBreitman

YouTube: www.youtube.com/LindaBreitman

RESOURCES

MIRACULOUS IDENTITY:
Unveiling Your Hidden Journey Curriculum

Featuring Teaching Components
- Miraculous Identity: Unveiling Your Hidden Journey
- Miraculous Identity: Study Guide
- Miraculous Identity: Video Series
- Miraculous Identity: Coaching Series
- The Real You: Believing Your True Identity
- The Real You: Activation Manual
- The Real You Video Series
- The Real You Identity Decrees
- The Real You Identity Decrees CD
- The Real You Video Sessions for Leaders
- Soaking In Your True Identity CD

These items can be purchased at:
www.LindaBreitman.com